Physical Conditioning and Cardiovascular Rehabilitation

Physical Conditioning and Cardiovascular Rehabilitation

EDITED BY

LAWRENCE S. COHEN, M.D.
Professor of Medicine
Chief of Cardiology
School of Medicine
Yale University
New Haven, Connecticut

MICHAEL B. MOCK, M.D.
Chief, Cardiac Diseases Branch
Division of Heart and Vascular Diseases
National Heart, Lung, and Blood Institute
Bethesda, Maryland

IVAR RINGQVIST, M.D.
Visiting Scientist
Cardiac Diseases Branch
Division of Heart and Vascular Diseases
National Heart, Lung, and Blood Institute
Bethesda, Maryland

A WILEY MEDICAL PUBLICATION
JOHN WILEY & SONS
New York · Chichester · Brisbane · Toronto

Library of Congress Cataloging in Publication Data

Main entry under title:

Physical conditioning and cardiovascular rehabilitation.

   (A Wiley medical publication)

   Based on presentations made at the workshop on Physical
Conditioning and Cardiovascular Rehabilitation, held May
16-17, 1979, at the National Institutes of Health in
Bethesda, Md.
   Includes index.
   1. Cardiacs--Rehabilitation--Congresses. 2. Physical
fitness--Congresses. 3. Exercise therapy--Congresses.
4. Heart function tests--Congresses. I. Cohen, Lawrence S.
II. Mock, Michael B. III. Ringqvist, Ivar. IV.
Workshop on Physical Conditioning and Cardiovascular
Rehabilitation, National Institutes of Health, 1979
   [DNLM: 1. Exertion--Congresses. 2. Exercise therapy
-- Congresses. 3. Heart Diseases--Rehabilitation--
Congresses. 4. Heart function tests--Congresses. 5.
Exercise test--Congresses. WG200 W9263p 1979]
RC681.A2P47   616.1'0624   80-230-58
ISBN 0-471-08713-0

Printed in the United States of America

10 9 8 7 6 5 4 3 2 1

Contributors

Chairman

Lawrence S. Cohen, M.D.
Professor of Medicine
School of Medicine
Yale University
New Haven, Connecticut

Co-Chairmen

Stephen E. Epstein, M.D.
Chief, Cardiology Branch
Division of Intramural
  Research
National Heart, Lung, and
  Blood Institute
Bethesda, Maryland

Jere H. Mitchell, M.D.
Professor of Medicine
Department of Internal
  Medicine
University of Texas South-
  western Medical School
Dallas, Texas

Michael B. Mock, M.D.
Chief, Cardiac Diseases
  Branch
Division of Heart and
  Vascular Diseases
National Heart, Lung, and
  Blood Institute
Bethesda, Maryland

John Naughton, M.D.
Dean, School of Medicine
State University of
  New York
Buffalo, New York

Albert Oberman, M.D.
Director, Division of
  Preventive Medicine
University of Alabama
Birmingham, Alabama

Ivar Ringqvist, M.D.
Visiting Scientist
Cardiac Diseases Branch
Division of Heart and
Vascular Diseases
National Heart, Lung, and
  Blood Institute
Bethesda, Maryland

Sponsor

Cardiac Diseases Branch
Division of Heart and
Vascular Diseases
National Heart, Lung, and
  Blood Institute
National Institutes of Health
Bethesda, Maryland

Authors

Ezra A. Amsterdam, M.D.
Professor of Medicine
Section of Cardiovascular
  Medicine
School of Medicine
University of California
Davis, California

C. Gunnar Blomqvist, M.D.
Professor of Medicine
 and Physiology
Department of Internal
 Medicine
Health Sciences Center
University of Texas
Dallas, Texas

Robert A. Bruce, M.D.
Professor of Medicine
Co-Director, Division of
 Cardiology
University of Washington
Seattle, Washington

James H. Caldwell, M.D.
Assistant Professor of
 Medicine
Division of Cardiology
Veterans Administration
 Hospital
Seattle, Washington

Rudolph H. Dressendorfer,
 Ph.D.
Director, Exercise and Pre-
 vention Program
Division of Cardiovascular
 Diseases
William Beaumont Hospital
Royal Oak, Michigan

Avery K. Ellis, M.D.
School of Medicine
State University of New
 York
Buffalo, New York

Lloyd D. Fisher, Ph.D.
Professor, Department of
 Biostatistics
University of Washington
Seattle, Washington

Charles K. Francis, M.D.
Chief, Division of Cardi-
 ology
Mount Sinai Hospital
Hartford, Connecticut

William L. Haskell, Ph.D.
Clinical Assistant
 Professor of Medicine
Stanford Heart Disease
 Prevention Program
Stanford University
Palo Alto, California

Herman K. Hellerstein, M.D.
Professor of Medicine
Case Western Reserve Uni-
 versity and University
 Hospitals of Cleveland
Cleveland, Ohio

J. Alan Herd, M.D.
New England Regional Primate
 Research Center
Southborough, Massachusetts

Michael C. Hindman, M.D.
Associate in Medicine
Duke University Medical
 Center
Durham, North Carolina

John O. Holloszy, M.D.
Professor and Director
Department of Preventive
 Medicine
Division of Applied Physi-
 ology, School of Medicine
Washington University
St. Louis, Missouri

John Hyde III, Ph.D.
Statistician
Biometrics Research Branch
Division of Heart and
 Vascular Diseases
National Heart, Lung, and
 Blood Institute
Bethesda, Maryland

Anders C. Juhlin-Dannfelt, M.D.
Department of Clinical Physiology
Karolinska Institutet
Huddinge University Hospital
Huddinge, Sweden

Veikko Kallio, M.D.
Rehabilitation Center
Turku, Finland

Francis J. Klocke, M.D.
Professor of Medicine
State University of New York
E.J. Meyer Memorial Hospital
Buffalo, New York

Steven F. Lewis, Ph.D.
Special Research Fellow
Department of Internal Medicine
Division of Cardiology
Southwestern Medical School
Dallas, Texas

Dean T. Mason, M.D.
Professor of Medicine and Physiology
Chief, Section of Cardiovascular Medicine
School of Medicine
University of California
Davis, California

Bengt Saltin, M.D.
August Krogh Institut
Copenhagen, Denmark

Roy J. Shephard, M.D., Ph.D.
Director, School of Physical and Health Education and Professor of Applied Physiology
Department of Preventive Medicine and Biostatistics
University of Toronto
Toronto, Canada

Richard T. Smith, Ph.D.
Professor
Department of Sociology
University of Maryland
Baltimore, Maryland

Henry L. Taylor, Ph.D.
Professor
Laboratory of Physiological Hygiene
University of Minnesota
Minneapolis, Minnesota

Andrew G. Wallace, M.D.
Professor of Medicine
Duke University Medical Center
Durham, North Carolina

Nanette Kass Wenger, M.D.
Professor of Medicine
School of Medicine
Emory University
Atlanta, Georgia

Preface

The major purpose of this book is to report the development and application of methods for evaluation of cardiovascular and other responses to exercise as a technique for rehabilitation of patients with heart disease. Most of the chapters are based on invited presentations at the Workshop on Physical Conditioning and Cardiovascular Rehabilitation held May 16 and 17, 1979, at the National Institutes of Health, and on commentaries based on the manuscripts. The discussions have been summarized and edited to place emphasis on the most important issues.

The current status of the field of physical conditioning and cardiac rehabilitation is reviewed. It is clear that in spite of substantial basic and clinical research on cardiac rehabilitation, the exact mechanisms by which physical conditioning affects patients with cardiac disease remain obscure. Furthermore, optimal investigative techniques are lacking.

Currently, several large randomized clinical trials evaluating the effect of supervised exercise programs on patients with cardiac disease are being carried out in the United States, Canada, and Europe. Analyses of the preliminary data of these investigations are included. Contributions have also been made by those scientists with expertise in newer techniques for evaluating cardiac function.

A number of recommendations are presented for appropriate areas for future effort. For instance, a thorough discussion is included on the results of randomized studies on exercise rehabilitation. A new collaborative randomized clinical study of the effects of clinical exercise programs on morbidity and mortality in patients with cardiovascular disease is not advised at this time. The experiences reported at the workshop from Finland, Sweden, Canada, WHO, and the United States showed high dropout rates in both the group randomized to the exercise intervention and the control group.

Furthermore, inadequate compliance for those continuing with the exercise program was reported. To have adequate statistical power, a study needs a sample of 3,000 to 4,000 postmyocardial infarction patients. Such an extensive study would require a disproportionate effort in relation to the type of data that would be realized. Conclusions would be based on the result of patients' experience rather than on randomization assignment, that is, essentially by observation rather than by analysis of the results of the randomization process.

The Finnish experience reported here suggests that the multiple risk factor intervention approach may prove to be ultimately more important in evaluating the effects of cardiac rehabilitation programs than in evaluating exercise programs in general.

Another recommendation set forth is that additional effort should be concentrated on small pilot randomized studies of specific subgroups of cardiovascular patients to clarify the value of training and other alterations of multiple risk factors in innovative programs of cardiac rehabilitation.

It is argued that the newer methods of evaluating cardiac function in patients within rehabilitation programs could better measure the effects of the different forms of intervention. Potential methods that look promising are gated blood pool scans and other radionuclide techniques and echocardiography. It is noted that there are particular problems with the ultrasound technique because at present it can be used only on patients at rest. However, an attractive aspect is that it offers the ability to perform multiple, repeated studies without radiation hazard. It also permits evaluation of cycle-to-cycle changes.

The need for additional behavioral studies involving the psychological and social aspects of rehabilitation of cardiac patients is identified.

Finally, the contributors note that since work in the area of cardiac rehabilitation is expanding, there is no need at present for a special grant program to fund research in this area.

The workshop recommended publication of the proceedings with special attention to the conclusions reached. In this way, the status of the field and ideas for potential research can be reported and emphasized.

We want to thank the chapter authors for their expertise, involvement, and cooperation and the invited workshop participants for their effective contributions to the deliberations and recommendations. We would also like to express our appreciation to the director of the

National Heart, Lung, and Blood Institute, Dr. Robert I.
Levy, and his staff for making this workshop possible.

We are grateful to Prospect Associates and its editors
Peggy Eastman, Karen Jacob, Merriam Lehman, and Judy
Sugar for their help with manuscripts and production and
to our secretarial staffs as well as Barbara Jordan,
Laura Simmons, and Cherilyn Anderson at the National
Heart, Lung, and Blood Institute for their assistance in
preparing the manuscripts. Finally, we wish to thank
our respective families for their encouragement and
patience.

Lawrence S. Cohen, M.D.
Michael B. Mock, M.D.
Ivar Ringqvist, M.D.

Contents

Physical Conditioning and Cardiovascular Rehabilitation

PART 1

PART 1

1
EXERCISE TESTS

Robert A. Bruce, M.D.

Assessment of cardiovascular function in relation to
physical conditioning and rehabilitation involves the entire range from minimal to maximal metabolic stress, both
before and after rehabilitative conditioning. This is
best achieved by use of standardized, multistage tests
which provide observations initially at rest, during in-
termediate levels of dynamic physical exercise, at symptom-limited maximal effort, and during the first few
minutes of recovery from such stresses.[1]

Arbitrary target-heart rate endpoints should not be
used;[2] instead, observations of the intensity and duration of the symptom/sign-limited exercise protocol, heart
rate, systolic and diastolic blood pressure, electrocardiogram for rhythm, rate, conduction changes, and particularly ST displacement, as well as elicitation of symptoms
and signs on re-examination of the subject, readily provide considerable information noninvasively.[3] This information should be compared with normal standards of
healthy persons of similar gender, age, and physical activity status in order to provide a reference for quantitative interpretations.

Comparative studies of three methods of testing of 26
normal men indicated that the highest values of maximal
oxygen intake, heart rate, and lactate were achieved with
a treadmill rather than with either a bicycle ergometer
or step test[4] (figure 1). A study of maximal oxygen intake of 51 healthy men who were tested by four different
protocols (figure 2) for multistage treadmill tests of
symptom-limited maximal exercise showed greater differences in total duration of exertion than in peak responses[5] (figure 3). The Ellestad protocol required
slightly less time than the Bruce protocol, but the
latter provides more appropriate gradations of speeds

3

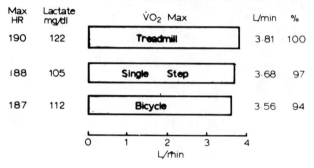

COMPARATIVE MAXIMAL EXERCISE PERFORMANCE
WITH DISCONTINUOUS TESTS IN 24 MEN
20-40(26 4)YEARS OF AGE

Max HR	Lactate mg/dl	V̇O₂ Max	L/min	%
190	122	Treadmill	3·81	100
188	105	Single Step	3·68	97
187	112	Bicycle	3·56	94

0   1   2   3   4
L/min

Adapted from Shephard et al, Bull WHO, 38, 757, 1968

Figure 1: Variations in maximal exercise responses in relation to method of exercise testing. (Reprinted with permission of Progress in Cardiology.)

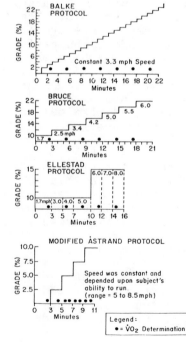

Figure 2: Differences in 4 protocols for multistage treadmill exercise testing. (Reprinted with permission of American Heart Journal.)

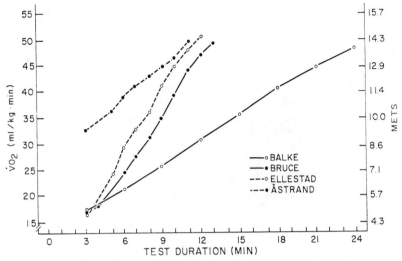

RATE OF INCREASE IN OXYGEN INTAKE IN FOUR STRESS TEST PROTOCOLS
ON 51 MEN, AGED 35-55 YEARS

Figure 3: Variations in aerobic costs and capacities of
the same men tested by 4 different exercise protocols.
(Reprinted with permission of American Heart Journal.)

and gradients of incline, ranging from strolling-walking
to jogging on an upgrade, which accommodates a broader
spectrum of healthy subjects and ambulatory cardiac patients. The aerobic costs, relative to individual VO_2
max and normal standards for healthy persons in general
community applications, have been extensively studied
and reported.[1]

It should be noted that although the physical workloads of stages I and II of the Bruce protocol are identical for all individuals tested, the relative aerobic
costs normally are greater in men than in women, and
especially in male cardiac patients (figure 4).

In regard to the methodological aspects, the duration
of multistage exercise by the Bruce protocol is highly
correlated with weight-adjusted oxygen uptake. In
healthy middle-aged men and women, the correlation coefficients are +0.92 (figure 5), and in ambulatory men
with heart disease the correlation coefficient is +0.87.
The relative aerobic capacity of an individual may be
derived from duration of exercise testing with the Bruce

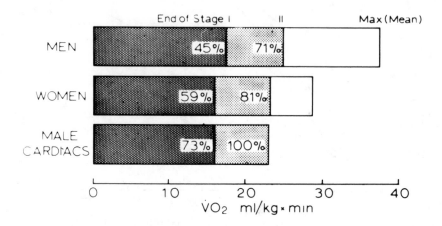

Figure 4: Variations in relative aerobic costs of healthy men and women and male cardiacs in relation to aerobic capacity. (Reprinted with permission of American Heart Journal.)

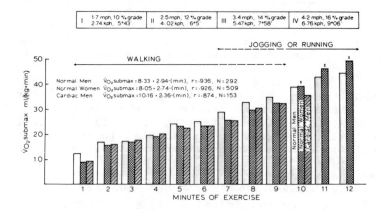

Figure 5: Comparison of weight-adjusted aerobic costs of first 12 minutes or 4 stages of Bruce treadmill testing protocol. (Reprinted with permission of American Heart Journal.)

protocol as a percent of average normal maximal oxygen uptake (figure 6) for a healthy person of similar gender, age, and activity status.[1] Likewise, the equivalent functional age of the individual may be estimated.

Nomogram for Men

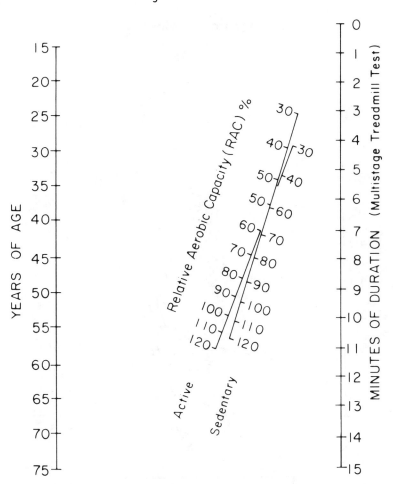

Figure 6: Nomogram for derivation of relative aerobic capacity of men. For example, 9 minutes exercise duration for a 45-year-old healthy man represents 80 percent or 90 percent of average normal maximal oxygen intake, depending upon whether individual is habitually physically active or sedentary. By extrapolating through 100 percent capacity, equivalent functional age is 58 or 55 years, respectively.

The complementary variable, functional aerobic impairment (FAI) or percentage of deviation from average normal VO_2 max also may be obtained with simple nomograms (figure 7).[1] For more exact estimates, the measured oxygen uptake may be related to age-predicted normal standards by use of regression equations. The percentile relationship of FAI for any given normal or cardiac patient may be derived from cumulative percentage distribution curves[6] (figure 8).

Nomogram for Men

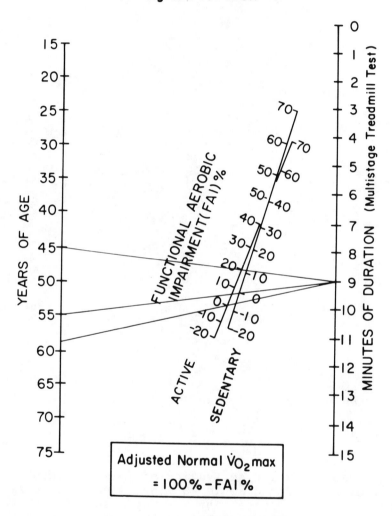

Figure 7: Nomogram for derivation of functional aerobic impairment (FAI) in men. (Reprinted with permission of American Heart Journal.) Lines refer to example cited in figure 6.

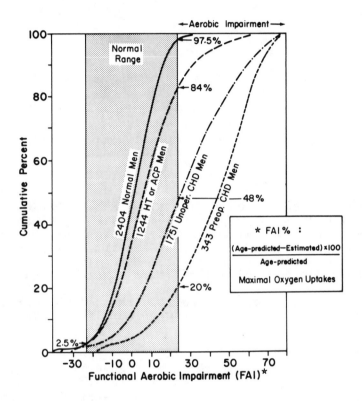

AEROBIC CAPACITY IN 5742 MEN

Figure 8: Cumulative percent distribution of functional aerobic impairment of healthy men and cardiovascular patients. Percentile relationship of any given individual may be derived from FAI. (Reprinted with permission of Hemisphere Publishing Corp.)

Despite marked differences in absolute value of aerobic capacity between men and women, the approach to maximal oxygen uptake in relative terms is similar, even for ambulatory cardiac patients with lower capacities (figure 9). Evaluation of maximal oxygen uptake reflects the functional limits of the cardiovascular system, but it does not reveal the mechanisms of its impairment. Of the three components of maximal oxygen uptake, namely, stroke volume and heart rate (cardiac output) and the

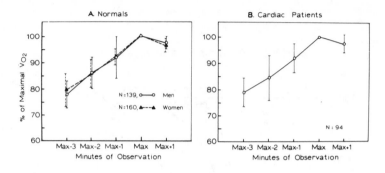

Figure 9:   Approach to maximal oxygen intake in persons
of different absolute aerobic capacities.   (Reprinted
with permission of American Heart Journal.)

difference between arterial and mixed venous oxygen con-
tents (A-VO$_2$ difference), only heart rate may be assessed
noninvasively.   Maximal heart rate defines the chronotropic capacity of the individual, and heart rate impairment
(HRI) may be derived to assess the percentage of difference from age-predicted maximal normal values.

Likewise, the percentile relationship of HRI for a
given individual may be assessed (figure 10).[6]   The

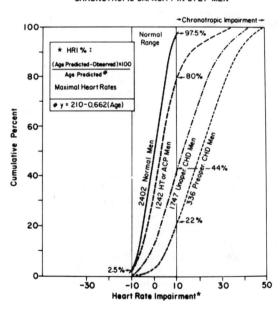

Figure 10:   Cumulative
percent distributions
of heart rate impair-
ment of healthy men
and cardiovascular pa-
tients.   (Reprinted
with permission of
Hemisphere Publishing
Corp.)

product of heart rate and systolic pressure (PRP) is a
simple parameter of left ventricular work which is highly
correlated with myocardial oxygen uptake,[7] even in the
presence of treatment with propranolol.[8] Accordingly,
the percentage difference between the observed product of
these two variables at maximal exercise and the age-predicted maximal normal value roughly indicates the magnitude of functional left ventricular impairment (LVI) when
neither aortic stenosis nor hypertension is present to
distort the pressure responses. Similarly, the percentile relationship of a given individual to his peers may
be assessed (figure 11).[6]

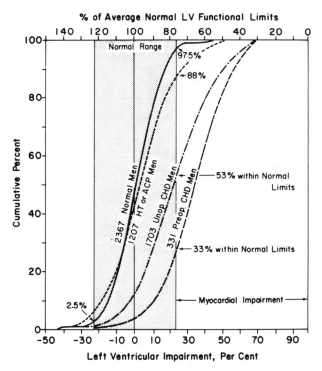

Figure 11: Cumulative percent distributions of functional left ventricular impairment, based upon percent difference from age-predicted systolic pressure, heart rate
X10^{-2} product. (Reprinted with permission of Hemisphere
Publishing Corp.)

Other mechanisms of cardiac impairment which may be identified by noninvasive testing include exercise-induced arrhythmias, conduction defects such as rate-dependent LBBB, and myocardial ischemia and/or dyskinesia. The prevalence of arrhythmias increases with age (figure 12). Similarly, the prevalence of ST depression also increases with age, whether or not heart disease is apparent (figure 13). There are two manifestations of myocardial ischemia: one is the subjective awareness of chest discomfort or pain of angina, while the other is ST depression. These manifestations may occur independently or in combination with each other.

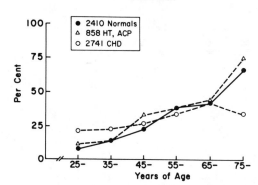

Figure 12: Age-specific prevalences of two or more premature beats in healthy men and in cardiovascular patients. (Reprinted with permission of The C.V. Mosby Co., in press.)

Figure 13: Age-specific prevalences of ischemic ST depression (one millimeter or more of horizontal or down-sloping) in healthy men and in cardiovascular patients. (Reprinted with permission of The C.V. Mosby Co., in press.)

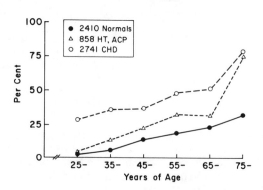

12

Visual interpretation of ST displacement is associated with considerable inter- and intraobserver variability. Furthermore, a systematic study of ST responses to maximal exercise of 58 asymptomatic men exactly 1 week apart also demonstrated limited reproducibility of the findings.[8] With visual interpretation by four observers, and computer analysis by two different methods, only 69 percent were placed in the same classification by the former and 75 percent by the latter method. Re-examination of the initial responses put 78 percent and 85 percent, respectively, in the same classification. Repeatability of classification by four observers ranged from 79 percent to 91 percent. The highest reproducibility was obtained by computer analysis of ST_2 at 1 to 5 min after exercise ($r = +0.94$).

Effective use of noninvasive exercise testing for routine clinical usage, primarily in office practice at the time of the initial clinical evaluation of middle-aged healthy persons and ambulatory cardiac patients, requires several prerequisites. These include preliminary clinical examination of the patient and history, and a resting 12-lead ECG to exclude persons who should not be tested because of contraindication. Informed consent for testing and followup surveillance evaluation are also important. Professional monitoring during exercise testing of healthy persons may be done by properly trained paramedical personnel when a physician has excluded the possibility of heart disease or other contraindications.

Testing of cardiac patients should be monitored by the examining physician, because this is often the most important part of noninvasive examination of the patient. In addition, he must be aware of indications for stopping the test in the absence of symptomatic complaints. In less than 2 percent of ambulatory individuals, testing is stopped when three consecutive ventricular premature beats occur, when there is a fall in systolic pressure below the usual resting level, and/or when an ataxic or staggering gait is noticed. Accordingly, there should be facilities for emergency treatment, including a ventricular defibrillator, oxygen, and cardiac drugs.

In rare instances in patients with clinically manifest coronary heart disease with marked hypotension, prolonged ECG manifestations of marked myocardial ischemia, or complex arrhythmias, the 12-lead ECG should be repeated after the test to exclude the remote possibility of myocardial infarction. The use of data forms to identify and to classify the individual before testing provides a simple but comprehensive method for recording observations. Terminals can be linked by telephone to a central computer to collect pertinent information. A summary of the testing observations is organized and immediately reported, together with interpretive data and prognostic information in relation to risk of primary or secondary CHD results.[10]

The broad spectrum of stages achieved in more than 5,000 tests of healthy persons and in more than 11,000 tests of cardiac patients is shown in figure 14.[5] More than 20,000 such tests have now been performed in the Seattle community without a single fatality; nevertheless, six cases of exertional hypotension and post-exertional cardiac arrest have occurred in men with severe coronary heart disease. Each was resuscitated by ventricular defibrillation without the complication of evolving myocardial infarction. Thus the safety of this particular protocol far exceeds that of coronary arteriography.

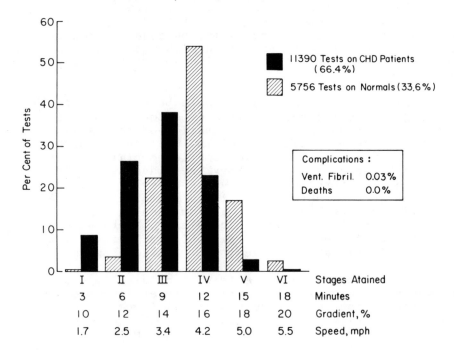

Figure 14: Distribution by maximal exercise stages attained in healthy men and in coronary heart disease patients.

14

In addition to the need for normal standards for interpretation of an initial test when individuals are retested at a later date, time-normalized longitudinal data are needed to indicate the usual rates of change of several variables in either healthy persons or in patients with cardiovascular disease (figure 15).[11] Furthermore, differences between sedentary versus physically active persons--as well as changes in activity classification in either direction--should be taken into account.

A low level testing protocol, requiring only 2 MET's for a strolling gait of 1.2 mph and 0 percent gradient, and increasing to 3 percent, 6 percent, and 9 percent gradient at 3-minute intervals and, if indicated, to 1.7 mph at 6 percent gradient for another 3 minutes, is becoming routine at the time patients are discharged from the hospital after treatment of acute myocardial

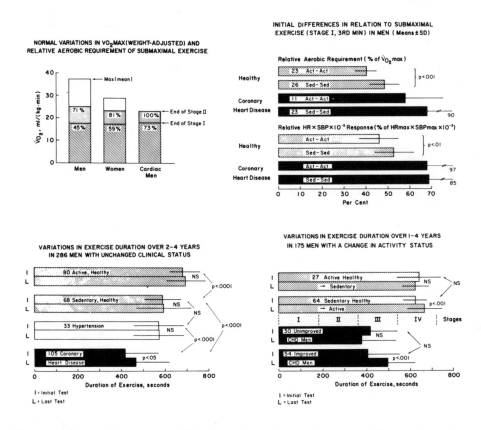

Figure 15: Reproducibility of selected variables at submaximal and maximal exercise and in relation to consistency or to changes in classification. (Reprinted with permission of Academic Press.)

infarction.[12] The highest workload requires 3 to 3-1/2
MET's, which is less than that of the initial stage of
the conventional Bruce multistage test (figure 16).[13]
Its purpose is entirely different, namely, to test the
reliability of the clinical judgment that a patient has
progressed sufficiently in convalescence to tolerate
casual, ambulatory self-care activities at home without
inducing significant cardiac symptoms or signs.

   The endpoint of testing is the <u>first awareness</u>, or
threshold, for any symptom or sign, especially tachycardia over 110 to 120 beats/min (varying inversely with
age, with even lower limits in the presence of treatment
with a beta blocker), arrhythmia, hypotension, or ST displacement of more than 1 mm (whether elevated, which is
usually more frequent, or depressed). About 80 percent
of patients with uncomplicated infarction can perform
all four stages for a total of 12 min without any of
these manifestations within the first 7 to 12 days;[12] the
subsequent incidence of disturbing symptoms after discharge seems to be quite low. This test performance also
alleviates the anxiety of patient and family that sometimes occurs with discharge from the hospital.

   For patients who manifest one or more threshold symptoms, such as angina, dyspnea, or fatigue or any of the

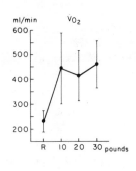
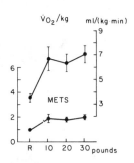
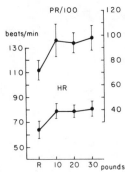
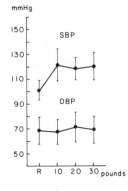

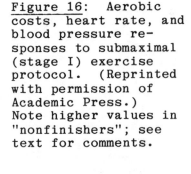

Figure 16: Aerobic
costs, heart rate, and
blood pressure re-
sponses to submaximal
(stage I) exercise
protocol. (Reprinted
with permission of
Academic Press.)
Note higher values in
"nonfinishers"; see
text for comments.

cardiac signs already listed, further observation and/or
treatment for 2 or 3 days and repetition of the same test
often reveals no threshold limitations. Hence this pro-
tects against premature discharge and the risk of unnecessary clinical relapses within the next few days at
home.

For the minority of patients unable to achieve all
four states of the low level test, heart rates are faster
and systolic pressures higher[12] (figure 17). These differences suggest greater sympathetic activity to compensate for lower cardiac output due to more extensive myocardial infarction and/or greater physical deconditioni-
ing. ST depression[14] as well as ST elevation (Bruce, unpublished observations, 1979) are important predictors of
cardiac morbidity and mortality within the next 6 months.

Figure 17: Differ-
ences in heart rate
and systolic blood
pressure responses
in relation to
ability of patients
with recent myocar-
dial infarction to
complete all four
stages. (Reprinted
with permission of
Heart and Lung.)

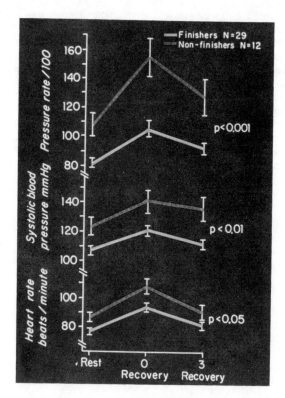

At a later phase of convalescence, ranging from 1 to
2 months after the onset of myocardial infarction, the
conventional "high level" multistage test of functional
aerobic capacity is useful to determine the maximal
oxygen uptake and to reveal some of the mechanisms of
cardiac impairment. This information provides useful
insights into the level of initial rehabilitative activities which can be safely tolerated and the possible

risks of arrhythmias, myocardial ischemia, or left ventricular dysfunction that may be encountered.

Serial exercise testing demonstrates progressive functional improvement, even in the absence of a physical conditioning program.[11] The amount of improvement and its time course[14] are also revealed by serial testing. About 80 percent of patients show such benefits; the others, who do not improve functional performance, reveal the need for additional invasive studies to ascertain the indications for and feasibility of additional medical treatment or aortocoronary bypass surgical treatment.

Noninvasive exercise testing is also useful to screen coronary patients in regard to the need or optimal time for invasive diagnostic studies, and, if indicated, surgical treatment to enhance survival for 4 years. Recent studies indicate that surgical treatment of myocardial ischemia does not improve survival, whereas such treatment in patients who manifest left ventricular dysfunction, noninvasively, are significantly benefited by revascularization when there are one or more arteries feasible for grafting[15] (figure 18). The predictors are the same as those that reveal a high propensity for sudden cardiac death in unoperated men with coronary heart disease.[16] They are cardiomegaly, peak systolic pressure during exercise of less than 130 mm Hg, and/or exercise duration of less than 3 min in the first stage (which requires only 5 MET's). The risk gradient based upon these three parameters of heart size and functional

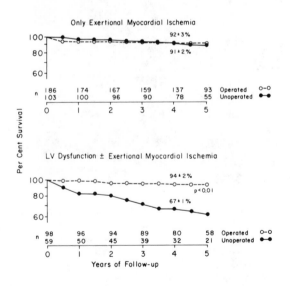

Figure 18: Comparison of survival rates of CHD men in relation to classification of exercise responses and to medical or surgical treatment. (Reprinted with permission of Circulation.)

limits of cardiac performance far exceeds that of exertional myocardial ischemia.[16]

One of the limitations of noninvasive exercise testing is the inability to ascertain the unknown precipitating factors responsible for inducing lethal arrhythmias or sudden cardiac death at a particular time in the lives and activities of coronary patients. Clinical observation and Holter monitoring often indicate the importance of psychosocial stresses as important contributory mechanisms at these critical moments. Another limitation is the inability to differentiate the remarkable amount of peripheral adaptation that accounts for the improvement in functional aerobic capacity with physical training.

Neither does noninvasive exercise testing reveal the gradual deterioration in stroke volume, even in the absence of symptoms, in individuals who regularly and vigorously participate in physical training for several months or a few years. Only invasive methods that directly measure both the cardiac output and the arterial-mixed venous oxygen difference (and especially the arterial oxygen content at maximal exercise) reveal the dissociation between cardiac function and progressive peripheral adaptations. For example, the mechanisms for the responses to physical training to treatment with propranolol are dissimilar, since arterial oxygen content during exercise is raised by the former whereas mixed venous oxygen content is lowered by the latter (figure 19).

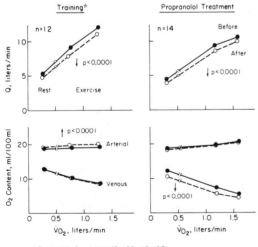

* Detry et al, Circulation 45:109-118, 1971

Figure 19: Comparison of changes in cardiac output and arterial and mixed venous oxygen responses to exercise in CHD men who underwent physical training or who were treated with propranolol. (Reprinted with permission of the American Journal of Cardiology.)

In conclusion, both low level and high level multi-stage testing of exercise aid clinical management of patients after myocardial infarction and guide the optimal use of exercise conditioning to enhance cardiac rehabilitation. Failure to use these methods increases the risks of suboptimal monitoring and clinical management of such patients.

References

1. Bruce RA, Kusumi F, Hosmer D: Maximal oxygen intake and nomographic assessment of functional aerobic impairment in cardiovascular disease. Am Heart J 85:546, 1973

2. Sheffield LT: Graded exercise test (GXT) for ischemic heart disease. In, Exercise Testing and Training of Apparently Healthy Individuals: A Handbook for Physicians. American Heart Association, New York, 1972

3. Bruce RA, Gey GO, Cooper MN, Fisher LD, Peterson DR: Seattle heart watch: initial clinical, circulatory and electrocardiographic responses to maximal exercise. Am J Cardiol 33:459, 1974

4. Shephard RV, Aleen C, Benade AVS, Divies CTM, di Prampero PE, Hedman R, Merriman JE, Myhre K, Simmons R: The maximum oxygen intake. An international reference standard of cardiorespiratory fitness. WHO Bulletin 38:757, 1968

5. Pollock ML, Bohannon RL, Cooper KH, Ayres JJ, Ward A, White SR, Linnerud AC: A comparative analysis of four protocols for maximal treadmill stress testing. Am Heart J 92:39, 1976

6. Bruce RA, Clarke LJ: Exercise stress testing. In, Proceedings of Starr Symposium on Heart Failure (Fishman AP, ed). Washington, DC, Hemisphere Publishing Corp, 1978, p 183

7. Kitamura K, Jorgensen CR, Gobel FL, Taylor HL, Wang Y: Hemodynamic correlates of myocardial oxygen consumption during upright exercise. J Appl Physiol 32:516, 1972

8. Jorgensen CR, Wang K, Wang Y, Gobel FL, Nelson RR, Taylor H: Effects of propranolol on myocardial oxygen consumption and its hemodynamic correlates during upright exercise. Circulation 48:1173, 1973

9. Trayler RE: The reproducibility of the postexercise ECG and PCG indices of myocardial ischemia. A thesis submitted in partial fulfillment of the requirements for the degree of MS, University of Washington, 1977

10. Bruce RA: Network terminal applications for cardiology. In, Proceedings: 1978 Workshop on Computer Laboratory Health Care Resources (Jarzembski WB, Rowley BA, eds). Lubbock, Texas Tech University School of Medicine, 1978, p 137

11. Bruce RA, Derouen TA: Longitudinal comparisons of responses to maximal exercise. Proceedings of International Symposium on Environmental Stress: Individual Adaptations, Santa Barbara, California, August 1977. Academic Press, 1978, p 205

12. Sivarajan E, Snydsman A, Smith B, Irving J, Mansfield L, Bruce R: Low level treadmill testing of 41 patients with acute myocardial infarction prior to discharge from hospital. Heart and Lung 6:975, 1977

13. Sivarajan E, Lerman J, Mansfield L, Bruce R: Progressive ambulation and treadmill testing of patients with acute myocardial infarction during hospitalization: a feasibility study. Arch Phys Med Rehabil 58:241, 1977

14. Davidson DM, DeBrook RF: Prognostic value of a simple exercise test three weeks after myocardial infarction (abstr). Am J Cardiol 43:353, 1979

15. Bruce RA, DeRouen TA, Hammermeister KE: Noninvasive screening criteria for enhanced four-year survival after aortocoronary bypass surgery. Circulation (in press)

16. Bruce RA, DeRouen T, Peterson DR, Irving JB, Chinn N, Blake B, Hofer V: Noninvasive predictors of sudden cardiac death in men with coronary heart disease. Am J Cardiol 39:833, 1977

2

EVALUATION OF VENTRICULAR PERFORMANCE BY RADIONUCLIDE TECHNIQUES

James H. Caldwell, M.D.

Using radionuclide techniques to assess right and left ventricular function during rest and exercise is a new and evolving area of investigation. Much of the initial development of a minicomputer system and software that permits such investigation was done at the National Institutes of Health by Drs. Bacharach, Green, Borer, Kent, Epstein, and Johnston.[1]

I will discuss the methodology of the two types of studies--equilibrium and first pass or first transit--currently used to assess exercise ventricular function, compare some of the technical advantages and disadvantages of each technique, and comment on the accuracy of the results and reproducibility. In addition, differences between the methods and the results of imaging during supine and upright exercise will be briefly discussed.

ECG gated equilibrium blood pool scintigraphy, which is based upon an imaging agent remaining in the intravascular space, will be discussed first. The two most common imaging agents are ^{99m}technetium-labeled human serum albumin or ^{99m}Tc-labeled red blood cells. The latter can be labeled either in vivo or in vitro and permit imaging for at least 8 hours after a single label. The scintigraphic images can be acquired with either a single crystal standard Anger camera or with a multiple, small-crystal camera such as the Baird-Atomic. Data acquisition depends upon an ECG signal being fed into a minicomputer, which uses the R-wave as a signal to begin acquiring scintigraphic events.

All the events occurring in the field of view of the camera and their x-y coordinates are recorded for a period of time predetermined by the computer operator--usually

30 to 50 msec--and then stored in the computer core as an image frame. Each subsequent segment of the cardiac cycle is similarly acquired and stored in sequence. With the next R-wave, the sequence is repeated, with summing of respective image frames (figure 1). This process continues until some preset count or time limit is reached.

R WAVE SYNCHRONIZED BLOOD POOL IMAGING

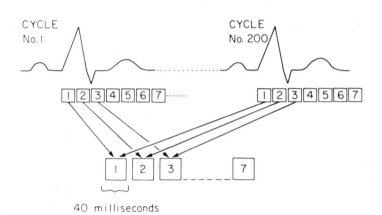

40 milliseconds

Figure 1: Gated blood pool imaging technique. Each cardiac cycle is sequenced into 40 msec segments beginning with the R-wave of the ECG. All the count data occurring within a given segment are then summed for all cardiac cycles and a composite image formed for that segment. (From Folland, et al, J Nucl Med 18:1159, 1977. Used by permission of author and publisher.)

After data acquisition is completed, the composite frames are linked together and are displayed on an endless-loop, flicker-free cineventriculogram of the heart. These images represent the activity acquired over 200 or more cardiac cycles at rest. Quantitative data regarding ejection fraction, regional contraction, and ventricular volume changes can be obtained by defining a region of interest over either ventricle and a background region as the ventriculogram is displayed on a cathode-ray tube. Time activity curves are generated from each region, and--using the assumption that counts are directly proportional to volume and independent of geometry--the ejection fraction and volume changes can be calculated.

By comparison, using the first transit technique for serial observation, such as before and after exercise or

24

other interventions, requires an imaging agent that is
rapidly cleared from the intravascular space. Those
most commonly used are the technetium-labeled sulfur
colloid or technetium pertechnitate. Either of the types
of scintillation cameras discussed previously can be
used, although the multicrystal camera is superior because of its higher count-rate acquisition capabilities.
For first transit studies, counts are acquired in either
a serial mode in which only the x-y coordinates for each
event are recorded or a frame mode as a bolus of activity
passes through the central circulation. Duration of
imaging is limited to the transit time of the bolus of
activity through the heart. The frames that were acquired during activity transit through the cardiac chamber being studied are then summed to produce a cineventriculogram usually consisting of only five or six cardiac cycles. Data analysis is essentially the same as
that used in equilibrium studies.

Table 1: Comparison of Advantages of the Two
Imaging Methods

Equilibrium	First Transit
Multiple studies possible	Short acquisition time
Acquisition during exercise	Anterior or LAO projec- tion
Wall motion with conventional camera	RV and left atrium ex- cluded
Not affected by arrhythmias	Upright exercise easier
Portable camera and computer	

   Turning next to the advantages and disadvantages of
each method, I would like to discuss them in the context
of how they might be used for serial exercise studies. A
summary of the advantages is presented in table 1. For
the equilibrium method, the images may be acquired during
exercise, not possible using the first transit method
and the multicrystal camera. Equally important, the
equilibrium method permits multiple, sequential studies
throughout exercise, whereas the first transit is restricted to a single measurement at rest and after maximal exercise. Serial exercise studies such as might be
indicated following drug intervention are easily performed

over a period of several hours using the equilibrium method and a single dose of radioactivity, again not possible using first transit techniques.

Additional advantages of equilibrium studies include (a) better wall motion analysis because of the statistically superior images, and (b) minimal effect by arrhythmias. With the relatively few cardiac cycles acquired by the first transit method, arrhythmias can greatly influence the results or reduce the image quality if excluded from analysis, whereas with equilibrium studies, the premature beats can either be excluded by the ECG gating mechanism or be averaged as part of the longer imaging period, and (c) the standard gamma camera found in most nuclear medicine departments can be used as is with only the addition of a minicomputer. In addition, portable cameras and computers can be used. The multicrystal camera, on the other hand, has not had widespread use--nor is it portable.

Advantages inherent in the first transit technique (table 1) include (a) a short acquisition time (15 to 25 sec), which allows the patient to stop exercise soon after developing symptoms, (b) acquisition of images in the RAO, anterior, or LAO projection, (c) structures other than the left ventricle, i.e., right atrium, right ventricle, and left atrium, are relatively easy to exclude from the images used for data analysis or can be analyzed themselves, and (d) it may be easier to image during upright exercise using first transit techniques.

Table 2: Comparison of Disadvantages of the Two Imaging Methods

Equilibrium	First Transit
LAO only	Suboptimal wall motion
Long acquisition times	Camera immobile
High spleen radiation	Number of studies limited
	Not during exercise (multicrystal camera)
	Marginal statistics (single crystal camera)
	Liver/spleen radiation

The disadvantages of the two methods are compared in table 2. For the equilibrium method, they are (a) relatively long acquisition times--1 to 2 minutes, (b) use of only the LAO projection for quantitative analysis, as this is the one projection that effectively isolates the left ventricle from the right ventricle and left atrium, and (c) when using labeled red blood cells, the spleen receives a relatively high radiation dose of 0.16 rad/mCi, although the total body radiation is roughly the same for a rest-exercise equilibrium study as it is for one rest and exercise first transit study.

In addition to being unable to perform more than a single rest and a single exercise measurement on a given day using the first transit method, other disadvantages include: (a) marginal counting statistics using the single crystal camera, (b) suboptimal wall motion analysis with the multicrystal camera because of inherently poorer spatial resolution, and (c) mandatory time between rest and exercise values of 15 to 20 minutes to allow dispersion and equilibration of activity following the first study.

The preceding has outlined some of the major advantages and disadvantages of both methods of acquiring radionuclide ventricular function studies. Next, the accuracy and reproducibility of radionuclide techniques will be reviewed, with the latter being a particularly important consideration for this conference in designing a longitudinal study to evaluate cardiac rehabilitation techniques.

When compared to the ejection fraction determined by contrast angiographic techniques, the radionuclide measured ejection fraction compares favorably in most recent studies.[2-4] The range of correlation coefficients has been between 0.80 and 0.95, and the standard error of the estimate has been in the range of + 0.10 ejection fraction units. Unfortunately, most of these studies have had only small numbers of patients. In a larger series of 50 consecutive patients reported by our laboratory comparing the equilibrium method with biplane cineangiographic volumes, the correlation coefficient was 0.83 with a standard error of 0.09 ejection fraction units.[5]

Similar results have been found by Drs. Andrew Wallace and Robert Jones at Duke University using the first transit method in more than 200 patients.[6] Most laboratories have found that the first pass method has a slightly better correlation with the contrast angiogram than does the equilibrium study, but this difference is not statistically significant. To further assess the accuracy of radionuclide techniques during exercise, we have performed simultaneous Fick cardiac output and radionuclide measurements during multistage supine bicycle exercise

to symptom-limited maximum. We have found that radio-
nuclide-derived cardiac output and stroke volume changes
were equal both in direction and magnitude to those
determined by the direct Fick technique (figure 2).[7]

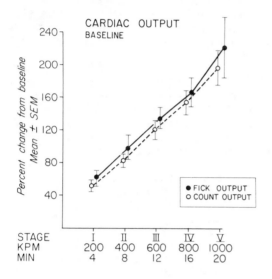

Figure 2: Compari-
son change in car-
diac output. A com-
parison of percentage
change from the rest-
ing value of cardiac
output during supine
exercise in normal
men. Cardiac output
was measured simul-
taneously by the Fick
technique and by the
radionuclide equilib-
rium blood pool
method. (Used by
permission of author
and publisher.)

The reproducibility of these radionuclide techniques is
at least as important as accuracy. Our experience--as
well as that of other reported series--indicates that for
a study done at risk, the intraobserver variability is in
the range of 1 to 3 percent for equilibrium studies and
2 to 7 percent for first transit.[4,5,8] The interobserver
variability is 3 to 5 percent and 2 to 9 percent for equilibrium and first transit, respectively. For serial
studies done either hours or days apart, controlled for
changes in HR, blood pressure, and intravascular volume,
the variability has been in the 3 to 5 percent range for
both methods.[8,9]

The reproducibility of the exercise ejection fraction has been less thoroughly studied. The largest
series reported using the equilibrium method has been by
the group at the Massachusetts General Hospital headed
by Dr. William Strauss.[10] Their experience indicates
that both intraobserver and interobserver variability is
in the range of 4 to 6 percent with serial variability
in the range of 5 to 7 percent. These results are similar to those of Ashburn and colleagues at San Diego,[11]
as well as ours. Little information is available on the
variability of the first transit technique during exercise. Serial variability results at maximal exercise
have not been reported, but Dr. Wallace and colleagues

have found the variability to be about 3 percent in a series of 10 normal patients.[6] All of these variability results using radionuclide techniques are equal to or better than the results reported for contrast angiography.

Exercise position as it relates to cardiac imaging is also an important consideration because cardiac output, stroke volume, heart rate, and blood pressure responses to exercise are dependent upon body position. These differences will therefore need to be addressed in designing a testing protocol. From the standpoint of nuclear medicine methodology, either equilibrium or first transit techniques can be used. The first transit method may be technically easier during upright exercise because the short acquisition times minimize the problem of patient motion. However, the opinion of the group of investigators with whom I am associated is that the other advantages and disadvantages of equilibrium and first transit methods discussed previously favor the use of the equilibrium technique.

The relative merits of supine vs. upright exercise for the evaluation of left ventricular performance have not been adequately evaluated. Studies of the sensitivity of these techniques for the diagnosis of coronary disease indicate equal sensitivities for the two positions of exercise when studied in separate populations.[1,12] No comparative studies in the same patients have yet been reported. In ongoing investigations in our laboratory, we have found no difference in the diagnostic sensitivity of the ejection fraction in a small number of patients (15 to date) exercised in both positions. The relative changes in end diastolic, end systolic, and stroke volumes are more pronounced during upright exercise, but change in a parallel direction to those during supine exercise.

Lastly, in reviewing some of the positive and negative aspects of radionuclide techniques in general as a way of evaluating the results of an exercise rehabilitation program, the following points should be considered. The major advantages are: (a) there are no anatomic limitations to performing the studies, (b) they are highly reproducible, (c) both visual and quantitative assessments of global and regional cardiac function can be made, (d) there are no geometric assumptions for volume calculations, (e) multiple, serial studies can be safely performed during exercise and other interventions, and (f) the same techniques can be used to evaluate right ventricular function. Limitations of radionuclide methods include: (a) suboptimal recognition of the ventricular chamber margins, (b) absolute ventricular volume measurements impossible at present using the radionuclide data itself, (c) the technology is rapidly changing at this time, such that methods chosen for a protocol might become obsolete during progress of the study, and (d) small amounts of radiation exposure to the subjects are involved.

In summary, radionuclide evaluation of global and regional exercise ventricular function is an excellent noninvasive means of serially assessing the effect of a cardiac rehabilitation program, and the equilibrium blood pool method is probably the method of choice. Two-dimensional echocardiography is the other major alternative technique, but it cannot be performed in a significant number of patients, and its serial reproducibility remains unknown.

References

1. Borer JS, Bacharach SL, Green MV, et al: Real-time radionuclide cineangiography in the noninvasive evaluation of global and regional left ventricular function at rest and during exercise in patients with coronary-artery disease. N Engl J Med 296:839, 1977

2. Folland ED, Hamilton GW, Larson SM, et al: The radionuclide ejection fraction: a comparison of three radionuclide techniques with contrast angiography. J Nucl Med 18:1159, 1977

3. Burow RD, Strauss HW, Singleton R, et al: Analysis of left ventricular function from multiple gated acquisition (MUGA) cardiac blood pool imaging: comparison to contrast angiography. Circulation 56:1024, 1977

4. Berger HJ, Gottschalk A, Zaret BL: First-pass radionuclide angiocardiography for evaluation of right and left ventricular performance: computer applications and technical considerations. Proceedings of Nuclear Cardiology Symposium, January 22-23, 1978

5. Sorensen SG, Hamilton GW, Williams DL, et al: R-wave synchronized blood pool imaging: a comparison of accuracy and reproducibility of fixed and computer-automated varying regions-of-interest for determining left ventricular ejection fraction. Radiology (in press)

6. Jones R: personal communication

7. Sorensen SG, Caldwell JH, Ritchie JL, et al: Serial exercise radionuclide angiography: Fick validation of count derived cardiac output in normal men (abstr). Am J Cardiol 43:355, 1979

8. Wackers F, Berger H, Johnstone D, et al: Variability of left ventricular ejection fraction by multiple gated blood pool imaging: comparison of normal and abnormal patients (abstr). Am J Cardiol 43:355, 1979

9. Marshall RC, Berger HJ, Reduto LA, et al: Variability in sequential measures of left ventricular performance assessed with radionuclide angiocardiography. Am J Cardiol 41:351, 1978

10. Okada RD, Kushner FG, Kirshenbaum HD, et al: Interobserver variance in the evaluation of left ventricular regional wall motion using contrast ventriculogram and rest and exercise multigated blood pool image (abstr). Am J Cardiol 43:355, 1979

11. Ashburn W: personal communication

12. Berger HJ, Reduto LA, Johnstone DE, et al: Global and regional left ventricular response to bicycle exercise in coronary artery disease. Assessment by quantitative radionuclide angiocardiography. Am J Med 66:13, 1979

3

RADIONUCLIDE EXERCISE STUDIES

Michael C. Hindman, M.D.
Andrew G. Wallace, M.D.

Cardiac rehabilitation is an effort aimed at improving
the functional capacity of patients with heart disease.
Like many clinical trials of primary and secondary prevention, rehabilitation programs attempt to control
major risk factors which are thought to contribute either
to the development or the progression of atherosclerosis.
In contrast to most of the current intervention trials,
rehabilitation programs emphasize exercise as an instru-
ment for therapy. This emphasis is understandable because of the close relationship between physical performance and rehabilitation.

The major purpose of this report is to examine the
hemodynamic response to exercise conditioning in subjects
with coronary artery disease. We hope to illustrate that
new noninvasive techniques make such an analysis practical and provide a basis for expanded studies to evaluate
the effects of exercise per se. An added objective of
this report is to suggest that the response to exercise
provides a useful technique to assess the benefits of
other components of a rehabilitation program.

Methods

This paper is focused primarily on 14 patients with
ischemic heart disease. Each subject gave a history of
angina pectoris, demonstrated new ischemic ST segment
changes on the electrocardiogram during exercise testing,
and had a greater than 70 percent obstruction of at least
one coronary artery documented by coronary cineangiography. Subjects with left main coronary artery disease or

an ejection fraction of less than 45 percent were excluded from the protocol described below. Other reasons for exclusion were hypertension which required medication for control, arrhythmias at rest or during exercise which required medication, and failure to adhere to the training protocol for a minimum of 6 months.

All 14 subjects participated in an exercise conditioning program. During the first 4 to 6 weeks, all exercise was medically supervised. After this initial period, some patients continued in the supervised program, while others exercised at home. The training program consisted of 30 min of walking or jogging and 10 to 15 min on a bicycle ergometer, 5 days each week. For the first month, the subjects walked and pedaled the ergometer at light (1/2 to 3/4 kpm) loads at a pulse rate below 100 beats/min. For the next 2 months, there were jogging intervals of 50-100 yards every quarter mile, or the load on the ergometer was adjusted to produce brief periods at a target rate of 15 to 20 beats/min below the level which produced angina or ECG changes. For the next 3 months, the duration of intervals of jogging and ergometry at the target rate was increased every 2 weeks with the goal of achieving 30 min of continuous jogging and 15 min of ergometry at the target rate.

Each subject was evaluated before and after 6 months of training. The evaluations were carried out without any cardiovascular medication for at least one week (i.e., propranolol and long-acting nitrates were stopped). The evaluations included body weight, lean body mass estimated by underwater weighing, resting blood pressure, a fasting serum lipid profile, exercise stress testing on a treadmill using the Balke protocol, and rest and exercise radionuclide angiography. Medications such as propranolol and nitrates were used as indicated during the training period.

The characteristics of other subjects and studies described briefly in this report are noted within the text.

Radionuclide angiograms were performed with subjects seated (upright posture) on a bicycle ergometer. All angiograms were done from an anterior projection using a Baird-Atomic System Seventy Seven multicrystal gamma camera equipped with a 1-in parallel hole collimator. Ten mCi of technetium-99m pertechnetate were injected into the external jugular vein through a 1-in, 20-gauge Teflon catheter. The radiopharmaceutical was dissolved in 1 ml of normal saline and flushed in with a bolus of 10-15 ml of saline. Precordial counts were recorded from the gamma camera at 40 msec intervals for 1 min after injection. The data were initially recorded on magnetic disk and then transferred to magnetic tape for

processing and permanent storage. Details of the data
processing have been published previously.

Time activity plots representing the change in counts
over the left ventricle were used to identify end systole
and end diastole, and data from three to six sequential
beats were summed to produce an average cardiac cycle.
After background subtraction, left ventricular ejection
fraction was computed from the difference between end
diastolic and end systolic counts. The perimeter of the
left ventricular silhouette was defined by the computer
at end diastole and volume was calculated using the area
length formula of Sandler and Dodge. End systolic volume, stroke volume, and cardiac output were then calculated.

To validate these radionuclide measurements, cardiac
output was measured simultaneously with indocyanine green
dye dilution curves in 18 normal subjects at rest and
exercise. Over a range of outputs from 6.6 to 21.3
l/min, the correlation coefficient between RNA and dye
estimates was 0.94. The correlations between left
ventricular end diastolic volume and ejection fraction
estimated by RNA and by left ventricular contrast cineangiography in the same subjects were 0.89 and 0.89 respectively. Reproducibility of the RNA measurements was
evaluated by repeating rest and exercise (same workload)
studies in 10 subjects 3 days apart. During exercise,
ejection fractions agreed within +4 percent and end
diastolic volumes agreed within $\pm\overline{2}0$ ml at the 95 percent
confidence level (table ').

At the baseline study, before training, radionuclide
angiograms were obtained at rest and at a level of exercise which produced ischemic ST changes on the electrocardiogram (most subjects also experienced angina). At

Table 1: Accuracy and Reproducibility of RNA Measurements

Variable	R Value	D $\pm$ SD
(1) LVEDV (ml) (contrast)	0.89	9.9 $\pm$ 5.1
(2) LV-Ej-Fraction	0.89	0.04 $\pm$ .04
(3) Cardiac Output (l/min)	0.94	1.24 $\pm$ 1.23

the followup study, after training, radionuclide angiograms were obtained at rest and at two levels of exercise. The first exercise study was performed at a workload on the bicycle identical to the pre-conditioning
maximal workload for each subject.

The second level of exercise after conditioning was
selected to produce a heart rate of 5 to 10 beats/min
above the pre-conditioning maximal heart rate. Exercise
was performed on a bicycle ergometer (Fitron, Lumex,
Inc.). The initial workload was 300 kpm/min and, after
1 min the workload was increased by 100 to 200 kpm/min
every 2 min. Exercise RNA's were performed during the
2nd min of exercise at any given workload. All data
were analyzed by a student t-test for paired data and
differences with P values of < 0.05 were considered
significant.

Results

The cardiovascular adjustments to exercise and exercise conditioning in patients with ischemic heart disease
need to be compared to those of normal subjects who undergo similar testing. Table 2 illustrates the hemodynamic responses to maximal exercise in normal young
adults before and approximately 6 months after training.
Before training, upright exercise produced an increase
in heart rate, cardiac output, stroke volume, end diastolic volume and ejection fraction. Training produced
changes during rest and during maximal exercise. At
rest, the heart rate was reduced, and diastolic volume
and stroke volume increased and ejection fraction fell.
During maximal exercise after training, the direction of
changes was similar to those observed before training.
However, maximal cardiac output was greater and this
increase was achieved by a greater stroke volume from a
larger end diastolic left ventricular volume with no
change in maximal heart rate or ejection fraction.

Data from the 14 patients with angina are presented
in tables 2 and 3. Before training, upright exercise
produced an increase in heart rate, stroke volume, and
cardiac output. In each case, maximal exercise was
limited by angina or electrocardiographic changes, and
the magnitude of the changes in heart rate and cardiac
output was considerably less than that in normal subjects.
Furthermore, these patients with ischemic heart disease
demonstrated an abnormally large increase in end diastolic
left ventricular volume during exercise, and in every
case, ejection fraction fell.

Table 2: Hemodynamic Responses to Maximal Exercise in Normal Young Adults Before and Approximately 6 Months After Training

	Cardiac Output (l/min)	Heart Rate (BPM)	Systolic Volume (ml)	End Diastolic Volume (ml)	Ejection Fraction (%)
Before training					
Resting	6.9 ± 1.1	74 ± 11	95 ± 21	132 ± 35	73 ± 6
Exercise	26.7 ± 0.7	185 ± 10	144 ± 30	169 ± 34	87 ± 4
After training					
Resting	6.7 ± 1.1	61 ± 7*	111 ± 26*	167 ± 40*	64 ± 7*
Exercise	31.8 ± 0.8*	181 ± 14*	170 ± 38*	197 ± 40*	86 ± 5

*Significant difference between pre- and post-training data.

37

Table 3: Effects of Training on Hemodynamics at Rest and at Exercise at a Similar Workload in Subjects with Angina

	Cardiac Output (l/min)	Heart Rate (BPM)	Systolic Volume (ml)	End Diastolic Volume (ml)	Ejection Fraction (%)
Before training					
Resting	5.2 + 0.7	81 + 9	65 + 11	112 + 33	61 + 16
Exercise	12.9 + 4.0	137 + 20	93 + 20	177 + 48	54 + 13
After training					
Resting	5.4 + 1.3	70 + 13*	77 + 18*	136 + 37*	53 + 15*
Exercise	12.9 + 4.0	126 + 24*	100 + 20*	194 + 39*	53 + 13

* Significant difference between pre- and post-training data.

The effects of training on hemodynamics at rest in subjects with angina are illustrated in table 3. Cardiac output was unchanged, but heart rate was lower and stroke volume was increased. Left ventricular end diastolic volume increased in most subjects and ejection fraction was reduced. The direction of these changes was similar to that in normal subjects, and appears to reflect a "training effect."

The response to exercise at a comparable workload in subjects with angina, before and after training, is shown in table 3. At a similar workload, cardiac output was the same after conditioning, but heart rate was lower and stroke volume and end diastolic volume were greater. Ejection fraction--which fell in all subjects before training--failed to decrease in most subjects after training.

All 14 patients were able to perform more work on the bicycle after training. When the workload was adjusted in each subject so that heart rate was the same or within a range of 5 to 10 beats higher than maximal before conditioning, every subject achieved a higher cardiac output (table 4). The average increase in "maximal" cardiac output was 4.0 liters, or approximately 30 percent. This increase in maximal cardiac output was attributable primarily to an increase in stroke volume (93 + 20 to 113 + 21 ml). The increase in LV end diastolic volume with exercise was comparable before and after training. However, ejection fraction, which decreased in every subject before training, failed to decrease in 10 of 14 subjects after training at the same or a higher heart rate.

Table 5 summarizes the measurable determinants of myocardial oxygen consumption at an exercise load which produced a comparable heart rate before and after training. Heart rate (by design) was the same or higher in every subject after training. Systolic pressure was higher after training in a majority of the subjects and the heart rate blood pressure product was higher in all subjects after training. Left ventricular end diastolic volume increased at maximal exercise after training in most subjects, but the difference before and after training failed to reach levels of significance. Ejection fraction, which decreased in all subjects before training, failed to decrease significantly despite a higher workload after training.

The 14 subjects who participated in this study of the effects of training on cardiac performance are a part of a larger group of patients with angina or myocardial infarction and documented coronary disease who have participated in our cardiac rehabilitation program at Duke University. Table 6 shows the effects of 6 months of combined exercise training (same protocol as above),

diet, and medication on several parameters of performance
risk factors in this cohort. Eighty-five percent of
those who entered the program have continued participation for at least 4 months. Among these subjects, the
median decrease in weight was 29 lb. The drop in serum
cholesterol after achieving a new steady weight was 66
mg/dl. Treadmill performance (measured in minutes using
the standard Balke protocol) increased by 6.9 min.

In addition to the above 88 patients, we have studied
12 patients with proven multivessel coronary artery disease and severe left ventricular dysfunction (ejection
fractions of 12 percent to 31 percent). In these patients, the cardiac response to exercise on a bicycle
ergometer was evaluated by right heart catheterization
before and 48 hr after beginning therapy with hydralazine
(50 to 75 mg P.O. q6h). After hydralazine, cardiac output was significantly increased at rest (4.8 ± 1.0 to
6.2 ± 1.3 l/min) and during exercise (8.0 ± 1.4 to $9.3 \pm$
1.3 l/m) (table 7). A-V oxygen difference was reduced
at rest and exercise. Before hydralazine, pulmonary
capillary pressure was 16 ± 6 mm Hg and increased to 31
± 12 mm Hg with exercise. After hydralazine, wedge
pressure was 11 ± 4 mm Hg and increased to 20 ± 8 mm Hg
during exercise. Thus, at the same workload and oxygen
uptake before and after hydralazine, cardiac output was
enhanced and pulmonary capillary wedge pressure was
reduced by hydralazine, despite a higher stroke volume.
These changes were associated with a lower systemic
vascular resistance, both at rest and exercise, after
hydralazine.

Discussion

This book is devoted to a discussion of methods which
are applicable to the evaluation of cardiac and other
responses to exercise as a technique of rehabilitation
in patients with heart disease. Exercise training is an
important component of a rehabilitation program, and
exercise testing is a useful method to evaluate the effects of training and other therapeutic efforts in such
patients.

The training program we have described in this report
adheres to the general principles of an aerobic conditioning program. These principles have been adopted to
also adhere to safety precautions which are advocated by
the American Heart Association and many investigators in
the field. Our protocol for conditioning differs from a
number which have been used by others. These differences
include the following: (1) training was performed 5 days
per week rather than the usual 3 days per week, (2) daily

Table 4: Effects of Training on Hemodynamics at Maximal Exercise in Subjects with Angina

	Cardiac Output (1/min)	Heart Rate (BPM)	Systolic Volume (ml)	End Diastolic Volume (ml)	Ejection Fraction (%)
Maximal exercise (before)	12.9 $\pm$ 4.0	137 $\pm$ 20	93 $\pm$ 20	177 $\pm$ 48	54 $\pm$ 13
Maximal exercise (after)	16.9 $\pm$ 3.0*	145 $\pm$ 23*	113 $\pm$ 21*	192 $\pm$ 62	55 $\pm$ 12

*Significant difference before and after training.

Table 5: Measurable Determinants of Myocardial Oxygen Consumption at an Exercise Load Which Produced a Comparable Heart Rate Before and After Training

	Before Conditioning	After Conditioning
Heart rate (bpm)	137 ± 20	145 ± 23*
Arterial SBP (mm Hg)	168 ± 26	175 ± 16
HR – BP – 10^3 (units)	23.0 ± 6.0	25.3 ± 7.0*
LVED-volume (ml)	177 ± 48	192 ± 62
LV-ejection fr. (%)	54 ± 13	55 ± 12

*Significant difference before and after training.

Table 6: Effects of 6 Months of Combined Exercise Training, Diet, and Medication

Variable	Baseline (Mean)	Change (Median)
Cholesterol (> 250) 18	251–410 (287)	23–167 (–66)
Weight (> 20%) 27	108–231 (167)	0–90 (–29)
Diastolic BP (> 90) 17	91–137 (97)	0–30 (–12)
Treadmill 88 (time/min)	2–12	2–17

Followup Interval (6-18 months)--88 Subjects with ASCHD.

Table 7: Effect of Hydralazine on Hemodynamics in Subjects with Multivessel CAD and Severe Left Ventricular Dysfunction (EF 12% to 31%)

	Cardiac Output (l/min)	A-VO$_2$ (ml)	S.V.R. (dynes-sec-cm^{-5})	P.C.W. (mm Hg)	LVED (ml)
Resting:					
Control	4.8 ± 1.0	7.5 ± 1.0	1,532 ± 366	16 ± 6	263 ± 8
Hydralazine	6.2 ± 1.3*	6.4 ± 1.2*	1,105 ± 352*	11 ± 4*	277 ± 8
Exercise:					
Control	8.0 ± 1.4	12.4 ± 1.3	1,008 ± 258	31 ± 12	288 ± 9
Hydralazine	9.3 ± 1.3*	10.5 ± 1.8*	805 ± 201*	20 ± 8*	289 ± 5

*Significant differences before and after hydralazine.

Hydralazine, 50-75 mg q6h.

Exercise, 300 kpm/min, O$_2$, uptake = 950 ml (± 63).

exercise included both walking/jogging and bicycle ergometry, and (3) the conditioning period was 6 months or
more rather than the usual 3 or 4 months. These are important considerations, because the cardiovascular effects of training in any subject are related to the intensity of the program and its duration. Because patients with coronary disease are very deconditioned and
can be advanced only slowly, the duration of a conditioning program is an important factor in determining the
cardiovascular response.

Our studies have confirmed the applicability of modern
radionuclide angiography as a technique to assess cardiac
and hemodynamic responses to exercise by a noninvasive,
reproducible and repeatable approach. There are trade-
offs between the gated blood pool imaging technique
utilized by many investigators and first pass studies
with the Baird System 77. Both provide new data regarding cardiac dimensions and ejection fraction that have
not been available during exercise with older techniques.
The first pass technique is well suited to studies of
maximal exercise, particularly in coronary subjects, and
it is more easily applied to studies of exercise in the
upright posture. We believe that upright exercise is
more representative of the types of activity carried out
during training and is the most desired posture in which
to evaluate the effects of conditioning and other rehabilitative interventions. Studies are needed which use
both the gated and first pass techniques to compare the
responses to supine and upright exercise and the degree
to which observations made in one posture can be extrapo-
lated to the other posture in patients with coronary
disease.

The observations described in this brief report illustrate that maximal performance and maximal cardiac
output can be enhanced by training for patients with
coronary disease and for normals. New data provided by
the radionuclide studies, which have not been available
with previous techniques, relate to changes in ventricular dimensions and ejection fraction. Training leads to
an increase in left ventricular diastolic volume and to
a decrease in ejection fraction at rest. In normals and
in patients with coronary disease, the increase in cardiac output with exercise and the further increase in
maximal cardiac output with training are attributable to
a higher stroke volume at any given heart rate. This
increase in stroke volume is achieved in both groups
from a larger left ventricular end diastolic volume.
Thus, the effects of training are not attributable solely
to a peripheral effect.

Perhaps the most significant observation in our
study is that after training, coronary patients failed
to show a decrease in left ventricular ejection fraction

at the same or higher workloads than those which precipitated angina, ischemic EKG changes, and a decrease in ejection fraction before training. Resting ejection fraction was maintained during exercise after training, even when two of the important determinants of coronary blood flow and myocardial oxygen consumption were the same or higher than levels which were associated with a decrease in ejection fraction before training. These data suggest one or both of at least two potential explanations. First, coronary blood flow or its distribution during exercise may be improved by conditioning. Second, some consequence of training not measured in this study may have reduced myocardial oxygen demand at the same or a higher heart rate, blood pressure product, and end diastolic volume during exercise. The effects of training on blood volume, on sympathetic activity and on velocity of myocardial shortening at rest and exercise in subjects with coronary disease warrant further investigation.

Although the major thrust of this report is aimed at exercise conditioning and the radionuclide method, we have included a brief report of the effects of hydralazine on the hemodynamic response to exercise for three reasons. First, because exercise reveals or exaggerates the physiologic consequences of coronary artery disease, it is not surprising to find that the beneficial effects of therapeutic interventions are more evident during exercise than at rest. In this case, the effects of hydralazine or pulmonary capillary wedge pressure were substantially greater during exercise than at rest.

Second, in subjects with reduced ventricular function at rest, the benefits of hydralazine on pulmonary capillary wedge pressure were significant even though no significant change of left ventricular volume was detected by radionuclide studies in the same subjects. Thus, in selected patients, radionuclide studies may prove to be a less sensitive method than more invasive studies to assess the benefits of all intervention.

Finally, it is evident from this study of hydralazine and from previous studies of nitrates and propranolol that pharmacologic agents enhance the capacity for exercise in patients with coronary disease. No systematic study is available yet to assess the role of concurrent pharmacologic therapy in a conditioning program, or the presumed effect. which would be to enhance the work tolerated during training and thus the cardiovascular responses to conditioning.

It seems clear that a large-scale multicenter trial will be needed to assess the effects of cardiac rehabilitation on survival and other important outcomes in subjects with coronary disease. The detail with which such

subjects are characterized before entering this trial
will be vital to its success. Assessment of the response
to exercise will significantly complement and enhance
other clinical and anatomic descriptions at baseline and
rest-exercise; radionuclide studies are a practical approach to this characterization.

A comparison of control and treated patients with respect to survival, infarction, etc., is vital to a complete understanding of the effects of rehabilitation.
Studies of exercise performance and of cardiac function
at rest and exercise, where the patients serve as their
own control, will also be meaningful in themselves and
essential to characterize the mechanisms of improvement,
if improvement occurs. Thus, any future trial of exercise conditioning should embrace studies which will help
to clarify mechanisms if the desired outcome is achieved.

In our study of a very small group of patients, we have
observed a substantial and significant improvement in
exercise performance, in the cardiac response to exercise
and in selected risk factors. We believe that, in the
design of a study to test the effects of exercise conditioning, it is important to allow time for the patient
to achieve a near maximal benefit from training. Certainly this is a matter of months or even a year in
subjects with coronary disease. Furthermore, in order
for any benefits that might accrue to translate into
effects on survival or infarction rate, the patients must
adhere to the program over a period of several years.
Thus, the rehabilitation team must be able to establish
a relationship with its patients which will last for
years, and the barriers (financial and otherwise) to
continuing participation must be reduced or eliminated.

SUMMARY: PART 1

Stephen E. Epstein, M.D.

Dr. Bruce, in his presentation, detailed the uses of treadmill exercise testing to evaluate patients with heart disease. He emphasized that there are several purposes served by exercise testing. In addition to its diagnostic uses, such testing allows assessment of exercise capacity objectively, and permits the elucidation of mechanisms by which exercise may be prematurely terminated, such as arrhythmias, ischemia, or exertional hypotension. Dr. Bruce also emphasized the importance of pre-discharge exercise testing following acute myocardial infarction. This type of exercise testing requires far lower levels of exercise stress than applied for standardized exercise testing. The purpose of such testing is entirely different from maximal exercise testing; namely, to determine whether a patient has progressed sufficiently in convalescence to tolerate casual ambulatory self-care activities at home without inducing important cardiac symptoms or signs.

For patients who exhibit angina, dyspnea, or fatigue, or other alarming signs of unstable cardiac disease, he suggests that further observation and possibly treatment for 2 or 3 days be undertaken before reconsidering discharge. Subsequent, "high level" multistage testing 1 to 2 months after the onset of infarction provides insights into the level of initial rehabilitative activities that can be safely tolerated. Dr. Bruce also described a high risk subgroup--those who had short duration of exertion, exertional hypotension, and increased heart size--who had a high cardiac mortality within the first several months following discharge. He presented data suggesting that these individuals have improved survival if treated by coronary artery bypass operation.

Dr. Caldwell succinctly summarized the relative strengths and weaknesses of different radionuclide techniques. Although there are pros and cons to both the equilibrium and first transit imaging methods, he appears to favor equilibrium studies. His reasons are based on the fact that 1) this technique allows for serial testing acutely, 2) measurements can be obtained during, rather than after, exercise, and 3) wall motion definition is better allowing more sensitive detection of wall motion abnormalities. The major disadvantages of the equilibrium technique are that the heart can be imaged only in the left anterior oblique position, long acquisition times (1 to 2 min) are necessary, and there is a relatively high radiation dose concentrated within the spleen. Correlation of ejection fraction with angiographic studies, and reproducibility of either radionuclide technique appears excellent.

Drs. Hindman and Wallace presented data on the applicability of radionuclide testing for assessing the effects of an exercise conditioning program. They demonstrated that training leads to an increase in left ventricular diastolic volume and to a decrease in ejection fraction at rest. In normal subjects and in patients with coronary disease, the increase in maximal exercising cardiac output induced by training is attributable to a higher stroke volume at any given heart rate. This increase in stroke volume is achieved in both groups from a larger left ventricular end-diastolic volume. Importantly, after training coronary patients failed to show a decrease in left ventricular ejection fraction at the same or higher workloads as those that before training caused a decrease in ejection fraction. This suggests that coronary flow during exercise, or its distribution, may be improved by conditioning. Alternatively, training may have caused a reduction in myocardial oxygen demand. In the discussion, it is pointed out that in other studies some patients have responded to training by increasing ejection fraction during exercise. Thus, the response to training does not appear to be homogeneous.

Discussion of Paper by Bruce

A question was asked as to whether a physician should be personally conducting every exercise test, or whether it could be carried out by a technician trained in cardiopulmonary resuscitation with a physician in the immediate vicinity who could respond within seconds to any emergency. Dr. Bruce felt that when a physician examined an individual and found no clinical evidence of heart disease, testing could be performed by skilled paramedical personnel. On the other hand, in the presence of significant disease, especially coronary disease, Dr. Bruce felt strongly that a physician should be present during the testing. He also emphasized the physician could gain far more insights about the patient's symptoms and physical findings by observing the patient under stress testing than he could in the office setting.

The question was raised as to whether ST segment displacement during an exercise test conveys information about prognosis. Dr. Bruce responded that in the presence of known stable coronary disease, ST segment displacement conveyed no important prognostic information. However, Dr. Bruce felt that low level exercise testing for the patient with recent myocardial infarction may provide prognostic information. Although the data are still very preliminary it was his belief that ST segment displacement in such an individual may be a sign of early morbidity and mortality. He cited four examples from his own experience of patients displaying ST segment elevation during exercise. Two of the four died within 3 months of recurrent infarction, pulmonary edema, or cardiogenic shock.

In response to another question Dr. Bruce reiterated that the workload he employs for patients recovering from acute myocardial infarction is low level. The patient walks at 1.2 miles per hour beginning at 0 percent grade. Dr. Bruce emphasized that the highest workload of this low level protocol is still lower than the first stage of his conventional protocol.

In response to a question concerning the relative risks of submaximal vs. maximal exercise testing, Dr. Bruce stated that as long as the patient had not had a recent myocardial infarction, and preliminary screening for acute problems was undertaken, and the patient was continually monitored by a physician, maximal exercise stress testing could be performed with safety and provide considerably more information than submaximal testing.

Dr. Bruce was asked whether formal pre-discharge exercise testing following an acute myocardial infarction serves any advantage above and beyond the observations a good clinician could make. Dr. Bruce felt that there were distinct advantages. In his personal experience he has seen patients whose physicians had been very confident the patient was ready to be discharged from the hospital, only to be surprised at unexpected pain, arrhythmia, or blood pressure changes occurring during low level exercise testing which were not present under routine ward activities. Dr. Bruce also emphasized that he does not perform such a test as a diagnostic study. He is interested 1) in defining the patient's cardiovascular

capacity and 2) if that capacity is impaired, in determining the mechanisms responsible for the impairment.
Thus, the goals are to provide the physician with insights into patient management rather than patient diagnosis.

Discussion of Paper by Caldwell

In response to a question asking whether it is possible to calculate absolute volumes from radionuclide
data, Dr. Caldwell replied that several groups are
working on this problem now. He believed that this
problem would be solved soon.

Dr. Caldwell was then asked whether he had important
concerns regarding the risk of low-level radiation. He
replied that the risk of the radiation is very minimal,
especially when compared to the risk of the underlying
heart disease most patients have who undergo this test.
Nonetheless, he realized it was the source of serious
concern for the patient. He compared the radiation
exposure from these studies with the recommended maximal
radiation dosage radiation technologists are permitted.
The equilibrium technique produces a total body radiation
of .1 rad, which is less than the maximal allowable
recommended dosage over a 3-month period. Dr. Caldwell
also indicated that the amount of radiation the patients
are exposed to is considerably less than that which is
acquired during standard right and left heart catheterization studies or coronary angiography. It is about the
same as the patient gets with an upper GI series.

Dr. Caldwell was asked whether he thought the appearance of regional wall abnormalities during exercise was
an important part of a radionuclide study. He responded
that if there is a regional wall abnormality at rest,
that abnormality remains during exercise. In his experience about a quarter of patients develop a new region of
dysfunction during exercise and he quoted a study from
Yale in which new abnormalities are found in about 50
percent of patients during exercise. He also felt that
the whole ventricle appears to enlarge with maximal exercise in patients with coronary disease; it was his
belief that the volume change may be an important part
of the information obtained during radionuclide studies.

It was also pointed out that end-systolic volume is
considerably increased after training. Some question was
raised as to the reliability of the measure of ejection
fraction as an index of contractility when end-diastolic
and end-systolic dimensions change so profoundly. The
point was made that the ratio of pre-ejection period to

left ventricular ejection time, which may be about .36 or .37 in cardiac patients before training after peak effort, will go down to .21, even though ejection fraction is not increased.

In response to another question, Dr. Caldwell answered that serial studies over months or years may be very sensitive in indicating underlying change in coronary anatomy. He has seen patients studied serially over a 2-year period who have developed progressive decrease in ejection fraction, which he believed probably reflected progression of the underlying coronary disease.

Regarding sensitivity and specificity of radionuclide cineangiographic studies in comparison to the exercise electrocardiogram, Dr. Caldwell felt the sensitivity of ejection fraction abnormalities at rest or during exercise in detecting CAD, was considerably higher than the sensitivity of the exercise ECG. He found sensitivity of the radionuclide test to be about 95 percent. He indicated that although specificity in his hands has not been as good as the exercise electrocardiogram, he acknowledged that the NIH group had reported considerably higher specificity. Dr. Caldwell stated that the reasons for the differences were still to be resolved.

Discussion of Paper by Hindman and Wallace

Dr. Hindman was asked whether there was any difference in the effectiveness of the exercise training program between those patients who continued the conditioning program under supervision and those who did it on their own. Dr. Hindman said that there were no differences between the two groups.

It was then pointed out that the increase in stroke volume Dr. Hindman demonstrated subsequent to conditioning was not necessarily a specific reflection of improved myocardial performance, but that peripheral adaptive changes, particularly those leading to a decrease in peripheral vascular resistance, might improve stroke volume by decreasing afterload. Another participant suggested that if such were important, it might have been expected to lead to an increase in ejection fraction, which did not occur during training in the coronary patients. On the other hand, Dr. Hindman pointed out that there were increases in end-diastolic volumes following training, a change which in itself might contribute to the observed increase in stroke volume without necessarily affecting ejection fraction.

Another participant related his experience with training patients who have coronary artery disease. His group found that some patients did improve the ejection fraction response to exercise after training. He also found a group that manifested a deterioration in ejection fraction. It was pointed out that the differences between his study and Drs. Hindman's and Wallace's might lie in the fact that they included patients with low ejection fractions, while Drs. Hindman and Wallace excluded such individuals.

General Discussion

Dr. Bruce stated that he believes noninvasive methods to be very interesting and exciting, offering much promise. He also wanted to indicate, however, that there is still additional information that can be derived from invasive studies. For example, he compared the effects on cardiac output and AV oxygen difference in coronary patients who had undergone a training program, to those who were treated with propranolol. With either modality of treatment cardiac output at all levels of activity diminished, and with each AV oxygen difference increased. However, the mechanisms responsible for the change, determined by invasive measuring, were very different. As a result of physical training there was an increase in arterial oxygen content and no change in mixed venous oxygen saturation during maximal exercise. He concluded there was a compensatory erythrocytosis of the bone marrow, which contributed more red blood cells. With propranolol, on the other hand, mixed venous oxygen saturation was reduced and arterial oxygen content unchanged, indicating that the increased AV oxygen difference with the drug is due to greater peripheral extraction of oxygen. Dr. Bruce felt this illustrated the need for both types of investigation, at least at the research level.

Dr. Caldwell stated that he did not believe we should think of the exercise ECG test and radionuclide test as competitive. He believes they are complementary studies.

He was also asked about the possibilities in the future of having a set of isotopes that will enable thallium and radionuclide angiograms to be performed together, so that perfusion and function can be assessed simultaneously. Dr. Caldwell replied that he felt it was potentially possible. He thought that theoretically one could inject thallium at maximal exercise during a first transit blood pool study; thus, as thallium uptake occurs, a thallium scan at maximal exercise could be obtained and the patient re-examined 4 hours later at the time of redistribution.

Dr. Epstein asked Dr. Bruce the question about the high risk subgroups he identified. This high risk subgroup is characterized by having an enlarged heart, exertional hypotension, and short exercise time. He asked Dr. Bruce whether this high risk subgroup could have been identified easily just on the basis of severe symptomatology. Dr. Bruce replied that the high risk subgroup doesn't necessarily have all three of those variables present. He pointed out that only one-half of 1 percent of the coronary patients they studied had the three simultaneously. His definition of high risk subgroup entailed an individual having at least two of these abnormalities. He did indicate that in some instances these patients are quite limited and recognized clinically. The objective measurements, however, did provide some way of quantifying how sick the patients were. He also has seen patients who, on the basis of severe symptoms, were felt to be at high risk but, after testing, were found to perform much better than anticipated.

Dr. Epstein then asked Drs. Hindman and Caldwell whether there was any noninvasive way to detect patients with left main disease. Dr. Caldwell indicated that in his experience radionuclide studies do not appear to offer that possibility. The data do not appear to distinguish the patient with single-vessel disease from the patient with left main disease. This response was in agreement with Dr. Epstein's experience with a small series of patients with left main disease. These individuals have an abnormal ejection fraction response to exercise; however, the response falls within the range seen in patients with single-, double-, or triple-vessel disease. Dr. Hindman had similar results, although the total series of patients with left main studied at any one institution is still too small for definitive statements to be made.

PART 2

4

PHYSIOLOGICAL EFFECTS OF TRAINING: GENERAL CIRCULATORY ADJUSTMENTS

C. Gunnar Blomqvist, M.D.
Steven F. Lewis, Ph.D.

Physical Performance Capacity

Human physical performance capacity has multiple determinants. The ability to perform any physical task is a function of (a) the capacity of the various aerobic and anaerobic mechanisms for transformation of chemical energy to mechanical work and (b) the ability to activate and control these mechanisms. Performance capacity has a significant (figure 1) genetic component.[1,2] Age and habitual level of physical activity are the most important of many physiological modifiers.

Clinical exercise physiology for the internist and cardiologist deals with aerobic exercise and the mechanisms that are involved in oxygen transport and utilization. Exercise that lasts for at least a few minutes and activates large muscle groups, e.g., various forms of locomotion, has the potential of imposing a greater load on the cardiovascular system than any other stimulus associated with the normal activities of daily life. This mode of exercise is particularly likely to precipitate symptoms in patients with heart disease and also is the mode upon which most clinical exercise tests and therapeutic training programs are based.

Work related to this review was supported by grants from the National Heart, Lung, and Blood Institute (HL17669, HL06296) and from the National Aeronautics and Space Administration (NSG 9026). Dr. Lewis is a Special Research Fellow (Cardiovascular Research Training Grant HL07360).

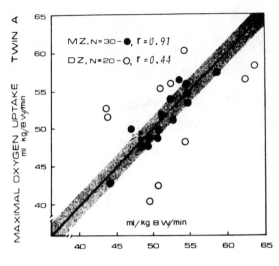

Figure 1: Genetic contribution to physical performance capacity. Maximal oxygen uptake in pairs of monozygotic (MZ) and dizygotic (DZ) twins. The shaded area represents the magnitude of the error of measurement. Measurement of maximal heart rate produce similar MZ and DZ distribution with linear correlation coefficients of 0.90 and 0.48.

From Klissouras[1] by permission.

The response to any form of physical activity can be modified by training. This review will deal mainly with the effects of training on the short-term cardiovascular response to dynamic exercise with large muscle groups. Important adaptations that primarily affect the ability to perform prolonged exercise (metabolic and thermoregulatory changes) or isometric exercise (changes in muscle mass and recruitment patterns) will not be covered, although they may have significant secondary circulatory effects.[3,4]

Oxygen Transport and Use

The principal links of the chain of mechanisms transferring oxygen from ambient air to the tissues are listed in table 1.[5] There is solid evidence from numerous longitudinal and cross-sectional studies that the lungs do not limit oxygen transport in normal subjects or in patients with cardiovascular disease.[5] The tissue diffusing capacity—which according to Krogh's concept is a function of capillary density, metabolic rate, and the capillary-tissue O_2 pressure gradient—may be altered by training and age. However, it is doubtful that the classical model is applicable to skeletal muscle,[6] and variations are in any case not likely to be of sufficient magnitude to explain the large interindividual differences in maximal oxygen uptake that can be demonstrated in groups of normal subjects. Therefore, the mechanism limiting aerobic work capacity is either cardiovascular oxygen transport or the capacity of the tissues, particularly skeletal muscle, to use oxygen.

The functional and metabolic characteristics of skeletal muscle have been studied extensively during the past decade. Links have been established between chemical and histochemical characteristics and physical performance capacity. Important changes related to changing activity patterns have been described in detail.[4,6-8] The presence of prominent adaptive changes in skeletal muscle has lent support to the hypotheses that (1) the peripheral training effects are primary and any changes affecting the central circulation are secondary, and (2) the peripheral oxidative capacity is the main determinant of aerobic capacity.[9]

There is no doubt that local adaptations have significant effects on the systemic response to exercise. However, several lines of evidence support the traditional view that the cardiovascular oxygen transport capacity is the limiting mechanism during exercise with large muscle groups. Quantitative estimates of the activities of various oxidative enzymes indicate that the potential of the total skeletal muscle mass to use oxygen exceeds the cardiovascular transport capacity.[8]

Studies in middle-aged men have demonstrated that training may cause significant muscular enzymatic changes in the absence of any effects on maximal oxygen uptake.[10] Furthermore, an increased oxygen content of the ambient air produces--in the absence of significant changes in

Table 1:   Principal Steps in the Oxygen Transport Chain

---

1.   Ventilatory transport

2.   Diffusion into blood

3.   Chemical reaction with hemoglobin

4.   Aortic transport (cardiac output x arterial O_2 capacity)

5.   Distribution of cardiac output and diffusion to sites of tissue utilization

---

Modified after Johnson.[5]

Steps 1-3 represent pulmonary transport.

59

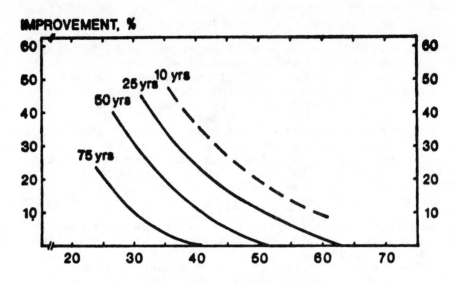

Figure 2: Relation between initial state of fitness and the magnitude of improvement in maximal oxygen uptake after training in different age groups. Data from 16 different studies, compiled by Grimby and Saltin.

From Saltin[15] by permission.

density and viscosity of the inhaled gas mixture--an oxygen uptake that is significantly higher than the maximum measured at sea level partial pressures.[11] Maximal oxygen uptake may therefore in normal subjects and patients with cardiovascular disease be viewed as an index of cardiovascular functional capacity.

Effect of Training on Maximal Oxygen Uptake

There is ample evidence (recently reviewed by Clausen[12,13] and by Scheuer and Tipton[14]) that dynamic exercise training programs of a duration of at least 4 to 6 weeks and based on exercise with large muscle groups will produce a significant increase in maximal oxygen uptake. The magnitude of improvement in normal subjects[15] tends to be inversely proportional to capacity

before training and to age (figure 2). An inverse relationship between the degree of improvement and pretrain-
ing capacity has also been established for patients with
coronary disease with and without angina pectoris.[16,17]

Other determinants of the magnitude of the response
to training include the intensity, frequency, and duration of the training sessions and the total duration of
the program. Attempts have been made to define the
relative importance of these characteristics, but a
consistent pattern has yet to emerge.[18,20] Intensity
may be the most important single determinant.[20,21] The
minimal amount of physical activity that may produce a
training effect has also been investigated. Heart rates
during training of 130 beats/min and a relative load
(defined as actual oxygen uptake as a percentage of individual maximum) of 40 percent have sufficed in some
series.[19-24]

As little as 30 minutes of relatively high-intensity
exercise accomplished during two to three weekly sessions
produced significant effects in one series of very sedentary middle-aged men, but a single weekly 12-minute session failed to maintain the improvement.[25] More information is needed in this area. It would seem particularly
important to perform studies that include a careful
evaluation of baseline activity patterns and a documentation of the training program in terms of the amount of
added activity. More data are also needed on the time
at which the various training-induced adaptations occur.
A phase-shift between the metabolic adaptations of skeletal muscle and the changes in maximal oxygen uptake has
been observed in man.[26] Animal experiments suggest that
changes in coronary flow patterns precede other circulatory adaptations to training.[27]

The general relationship between the amount of training (intensity, frequency, duration of sessions and
total duration of the program) and the degree of the
improvement seems to be defined by a sigmoid stimulus-
response curve.[25] There is an apparent threshold level
which probably is a function of peak habitual levels of
activity between training, and returns rapidly diminish
once a certain stimulus level has been reached.

Specific Circulatory Effects of Training

The overall cardiovascular effects of training may be
viewed in terms of a rearranged Fick equation where Oxygen Uptake = Stroke Volume x Heart Rate x A-VO$_2$ difference. Cross-sectional comparisons of healthy individuals
with markedly different maximal oxygen uptakes indicate

that the variations can be accounted for largely by differences in maximal stroke volume and cardiac output. Variations in total A-VO$_2$ difference and maximal heart rate are quantitatively far less important.[3,5,12-15]

Any training-induced increase in maximal oxygen uptake in normal subjects is likely to be associated with an increase in maximal stroke volume and cardiac output. Maximal heart rate is either unchanged or only slightly lower after training, but a decreased heart rate at any given submaximal level of oxygen uptake is the most consistent of all training effects.[3,5,12-15] A few investigators have reported decreased submaximal cardiac output after training[28-30] but most series have shown no change in the relation between submaximal oxygen uptake and cardiac output.[12-15,31,32]

The maximal A-VO$_2$ difference in subjects with normal arterial O$_2$ content is a function of the capacity to extract oxygen and to redistribute cardiac output by reflex vasoconstriction in inactive tissues and metabolically induced vasodilation in muscle. The A-VO$_2$ difference is wider after training in normal young men[31] but does not change in women[21] or middle-aged men.[33] The reasons for this discrepancy are not apparent. Data relating to oxidative capacity, blood flow, and vascularity of skeletal muscle provide no clues. Training can induce an increase in the in vitro activity of oxidative enzymes in most subjects irrespective of age and sex,[8] but absolute levels tend to be lower in women than in men.[6]

The number of capillaries per muscle fiber also increases with training and increasing maximal oxygen uptake and decreases with age. However, the capillary/fiber ratio is similar at comparable levels of maximal oxygen uptake in men and women.[6] Furthermore, there is no evidence for any age- or sex-related impairment of vasoconstriction in inactive tissues during exercise.[3]

Patients with coronary disease share with normal subjects the training-induced relative bradycardia at submaximal levels of exercise, but the stroke volume changes are in most series small or nonexistent.[13,14,17] Cardiac output is often reduced at submaximal workloads and the A-VO$_2$ difference is wider.[13,14,16,17,34] The net effect is less cardiac work at any submaximal level of total body work and a decreased likelihood that a given physical task will produce angina pectoris and other manifestations of myocardial ischemia. A reduction in cardiac work also benefits patients who do not have angina pectoris and who appear to be limited by systemic rather than by regional or myocardial oxygen transport.[35] The effects of myocardial ischemia on pump function after training are likely to become manifest at a higher total body workload.

The principal features of the cardiovascular response to training and inactivity in normal subjects were well documented by the mid-1960's.[28-32] More recent studies have demonstrated that the gross cardiovascular changes are produced by a complex set of interacting central and peripheral mechanisms operating at multiple levels, e.g., structural, metabolic, and regulatory.

Cardiac Dimensions

There is a large body of older, mainly German and Scandinavian literature on the relationship between heart size and physical performance in athletes and normal subjects. In general, total heart size--as estimated from bi-plane radiographs--has been found in cross-sectional studies to correlate closely with maximal oxygen uptake, cardiac output, and stroke volume.[36-40] The results from longitudinal series are less consistent; they range from a close correlation between changes in maximal oxygen uptake and stroke volume and total heart size in young normal subjects[31] to no correlation in middle-aged men.[25,33] Activity-related changes in cardiac dimensions can develop within weeks.[31,41] On the other hand, former endurance athletes, including young women, who have trained intensely over several years and later adopted a level of relative inactivity, maintain a large heart size.[30,36,39,42]

Studies based on echocardiographic[41,43-46] and radio-nuclear techniques[47] have generated specific and detailed dimensional data. It has been suggested that endurance training, i.e., a chronic volume load, causes an increase in left ventricular end-diastolic volume without any changes in wall thickness, whereas isometric exercise, a pressure load, produces an increased wall thickness without any change in left ventricular volume.[43] Recent studies[46] indicate that both dynamic and isometric training cause an increase in absolute left ventricular mass but only endurance training increases mass normalized with respect to lean body mass. The left ventricular mass/volume ratio remains normal. Echocardiographic[48] and radionuclear studies[49] have also documented increased left ventricular dimensions after training in patients with coronary disease.

Myocardial Perfusion

There is experimental evidence for a training-induced increase in the size of the coronary vascular bed.[14,50]

The extent to which the increase exceeds the increase in
mass in the normal heart remains to be determined, but it
is unlikely that myocardial perfusion is a primary limiting factor in normal subjects. Direct measurements in
man have demonstrated that a linear relationship between
coronary flow and myocardial work is maintained also
during maximal and near-maximal total body workloads.[51,52]

Studies in several different experimental models with
surgically induced coronary artery lesions have shown
favorable training effects on coronary flow patterns.[14,53]
The human data are less conclusive. Coronary angiography
before and after training has failed to demonstrate any
development of major collateral vessels.[54,55] Many patients with angina pectoris are nevertheless able to
tolerate a higher rate pressure product (RPP) during exercise after training.[55] This is consistent with improved
myocardial oxygen supply since the RPP, i.e., the product
of heart rate and systolic arterial pressure, is the
peripheral determinant of myocardial oxygen demand and
of coronary flow in normal subjects.[52] However, the RPP
threshold of myocardial ischemia during atrial pacing[55]
is unaffected by training, which virtually rules out
major training effects on the anatomy and maximal conductance of the coronary vasculature.

Thus, the apparent change in ischemic threshold is
likely to be due to specific functional adaptations that
alter the relationship between hemodynamic work and myocardial oxygen demand or to regulatory changes that improve myocardial oxygen supply during exercise but not
during other forms of stress. Recent studies, including
scintigraphic measurements of left ventricular dimensions[49] in symptomatic patients with coronary disease,
provide some support for the second of these mechanisms.
Wallace et al.[49] reported an increased RPP at peak exercise levels after training. Left ventricular end-
diastolic volume, which is a major determinant of myocardial oxygen demand unaccounted for by the RPP, also
increased significantly after training, whereas left
ventricular ejection fraction decreased at rest and was
unchanged during exercise.

Ventricular Function

It seems likely that an increase in left ventricular
dimensions contributes significantly to the improved pump
performance after training--both in normal subjects and
in patients with coronary disease. Further studies are
necessary to define the relative importance of changes in
myocardial perfusion, and ventricular mass compared to

other determinants of cardiac performance, e.g., intrinsic contractile state, autonomic cardiac activity, and changes in preload and afterload.

Experimental studies have demonstrated cardiac biochemical adaptations to training which generally are less prominent than the changes in skeletal muscle and affect the utilization rather than the formation of high-energy phosphate bonds.[14] Studies based on isolated perfused and working heart preparations suggest improved mechanical myocardial performance and relative resistance to ischemia after training,[56] but results from papillary muscle preparations[57] are highly variable and inconclusive.

Human data are difficult to evaluate due to training-induced changes in heart rate, afterload, and preload. Longitudinal and cross-sectional echocardiographic studies[41,43-46] have provided no convincing evidence for physiologically significant changes in intrinsic contractile properties. However, training may improve myocardial performance by enhancing the contractile response to beta-adrenergic stimulation. Support for this mechanism can be derived from experimental studies.[27,58,59] Corresponding human data are not available.

Afterload reduction due to increased conductance of working skeletal muscle may account for a major portion of the increase in maximal stroke volume and cardiac output in normal subjects after training.[12] The exact mechanisms remain controversial, but include an increased vascularity of skeletal muscle.[14,15]

A large amount of data from cross-sectional and longitudinal studies have demonstrated a strong correlation (figure 3) between total systemic conductance and maximal oxygen uptake.[12] Cardiac output may reach 40 liters/min in a champion endurance-athlete who is likely to have a lower mean arterial pressure during maximal work than a sedentary middle-aged individual with a maximal cardiac output of 10 liters/min, i.e., data representing a better than 4-fold difference with respect to maximal conductance. Physical training generally produces a lower arterial pressure at rest but blood pressures during exercise in young normal subjects do not change significantly.[12,14,31] Older and unfit subjects are more likely to show a blood pressure reduction, as are patients with hypertension or coronary disease.[12-14]

There are only limited data on the effect of training on venous return and preload. A reduction in systemic vascular resistance would itself have a favorable effect on venous return, according to Guyton's model.[60] Acute blood volume expansion has little or no effect on maximal performance[61] unless the oxygen-carrying capacity of arterial blood is increased.[62] However, there is some evidence to suggest an increased preload during exercise after training. Changes in physical activity and maximal oxygen uptake are paralleled by small but significant changes in total blood volume,[31] usually without major changes in hemoglobin concentration or hematocrit. Well-trained athletes have higher pulmonary arterial wedge pressures during supine exercise than sedentary normal subjects.[63]

Both right and left ventricular filling pressures during exercise increase with age, and very high wedge pressures have been recorded in elderly men with high maximal

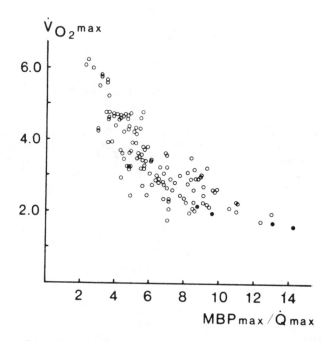

Figure 3: Maximal oxygen uptake as a function of total systemic peripheral resistance, expressed as the ratio mean arterial blood pressure/cardiac output during maximal work (MBP_{max}/Q_{max}). Open circles represent individual measurements in normal young and middle-aged men and women and in patients with coronary heart disease or hypertension. Closed circles denote group mean values. The distribution is defined by the regression equation: $y = 11.8/x^{0.72}$ where y is maximal oxygen uptake in liters/min and x the ratio mean arterial blood pressure (mmHg)/cardiac output (liters/min). The correlation coefficient is 0.87.

From Clausen[12] by permission.

oxygen uptake and cardiac output.[64] The improved pump
performance after training in patients with coronary
disease also appears to be associated with higher left
ventricular filling pressures and larger left ventricular
end-diastolic volumes.[48,49]

Regulatory and Peripheral Training Effects

Several features of the response to progressively
heavier exercise are normally more closely related to
relative than to absolute workload.[3,40] Substrate utilization (fat versus carbohydrates), pattern of recruitment
of specific fiber types, heart rate, respiratory rate,
total A-V O_2 difference and the degree of vasoconstriction in the renal and hepatosplanchnic circulations can
all be related to relative load. An increased maximal
oxygen uptake therefore means that work at any given absolute submaximal level can be performed more economical-
ly. The cost of oxygen transport is reduced, i.e., myocardial and respiratory work is lower, and the hemodynamic and metabolic reserve capacity is enhanced. The
exact mechanisms that link responses to relative load
have not been clearly defined. The response to exercise
is affected by multiple reflex mechanisms with receptors
in skeletal muscle and in the central circulation.

There are also links between the motor cortex and regulatory cardiovascular centers, providing a matrix for
"central command" and "cortical radiation."[65,66] Chemoreceptors sensing the condition of mixed venous blood
would provide a means of monitoring relative load, but
attempts to isolate such receptors have failed. Studies
of dynamic and isometric exercise, including training
studies and the use of arm exercise and one-legged exercise, have documented that local adaptations significantly alter the systemic hemodynamic response.[12,13,26]

The metabolic state of the muscle--which is a function
of relative load--probably determines impulse traffic in
the muscle afferents. Stimulation of muscle receptors is
a major determinant of the cardiovascular response to
isometric exercise,[65,66] and there are also data supporting an important role in dynamic exercise.[67] The separa-
tion and identification of training effects on central
command or cortical radiation, muscle reflexes, and reflexes originating in the carotid and intrathoracic baro-
and chemoreceptors, remains a key area of investigation
in exercise physiology.

The complexity of the regulatory changes that are induced by training is well illustrated by the effects on
heart rate. The normal heart rate response to exercise

is mediated by a combination of vagal withdrawal and beta-adrenergic stimulation. The essentially linear relationship between heart rate during exercise and relative load is not altered by training or deconditioning,[31] but sinus bradycardia at rest and decreased heart rate at any absolute level of submaximal oxygen uptake are the hallmark of a cardiovascular training effect. The bradycardia is usually associated with an increase in stroke volume, but the relationship is not obligatory or causal. Training-induced bradycardia often occurs in patients with coronary disease in the absence of any stroke volume changes.[12,14,17]

The combined results from normal and abnormal human subjects and various experimental preparations[14,68] have provided indirect evidence for decreased adrenergic activity after training. Plasma levels of epinephrine during exercise are lower both in normal subjects and in patients with coronary disease.[69] There is little or no change in norepinephrine levels. Data on myocardial levels of catecholamines are conflicting.[68] Responses to beta-adrenergic stimulation and blockade in various models have also been inconsistent. Less epinephrine may be present at cardiac receptor sites after training, but the sensitivity of the $beta_1$ receptors may be increased.[68] There is more agreement on the training effects on the parasympathetic system, with considerable evidence relating the bradycardia to increased availability of acetylcholine at the cardiac receptor level,[68] perhaps due to an increased synthesis.[70]

Several studies have also demonstrated a significant non-autonomic component of the training-induced bradycardia, i.e., a decrease in intrinsic sinus node rate as measured after combined vagal and beta-adrenergic blockade.[71] The exact mechanisms are not known. However, all cardiac pacemakers respond to stretch with an increased rate of discharge,[72] and it is tempting to speculate that the hemodynamic volume load associated with training may produce a stress relaxation phenomenon in the sinus node.

The exercise-induced reduction of blood flow to tissues that are metabolically less active than skeletal muscle, i.e., the kidneys, the liver, and the splanchnic organs, is strongly related to relative load[3,12,13] and to the level of adrenergic stimulation. The training effects on blood flow patterns parallel the effects on heart rate, i.e., the inverse relationship between relative load and flow remains essentially the same after training, but perfusion is improved at any absolute submaximal level of oxygen uptake.[12,13]

Thus, autonomic function is a major determinant of the acute response to exercise, and training induces major adaptive changes. Nevertheless, there is strong evidence that training effects can also be produced in the absence of an intact autonomic nervous system. Significant changes in maximal oxygen uptake and hemodynamic responses have been observed in patients with coronary disease[73],[74] and normal subjects[75] who--during endurance training--were treated with moderately high oral doses of beta-blocking agents. Training effects have also been induced in a variety of experimental animal models[14],[68] with significantly altered autonomic and metabolic regulation (unilateral vagotomy, immunological sympathectomy, diencephalic lesions, thyroidectomy, adrenalectomy, hypophysectomy, genetic hypertension).

This is an area that needs further exploration to provide more insight into basic mechanisms and to identify harmful and beneficial interactions between training and autonomic agonists and antagonists. For example, there is evidence for differential inotropic and chronotropic responses to acute stimulation of cardiac $beta_1$ receptors.[76] Available data suggest decreased chronotropic and increased inotropic sensitivity after training,[14],[27],[58],[59],[68] but the effects on different subsets of receptors have not been systemically studied. The role of beta-adrenergic mechanisms as determinants of the acute response to exercise is poorly understood, and even less is known about training effects.[77] It would also be important to establish the extent to which the autonomic and metabolic conditions that characterize large muscle exercise at moderate and high intensities are essential to the achievement of classical circulatory training effects. Preliminary data suggest that peripheral training effects, including the enzymatic adaptation in skeletal muscle, can be achieved at very low levels of myocardial and total body work by sequential high-intensity dynamic exercise training of small muscle groups (Gaffney, Grimby, et al., personal communication).

In summary, this review has demonstrated that physical training produces important adaptive changes in the circulatory system, mediated by multiple and interlocking central and peripheral mechanisms. The principal training effects include an increased capacity for oxygen transport in normal subjects and a more favorable relationship between cardiac and total body work in patients with coronary disease.

References

1. Klissouras V: Heritability of adaptive variation. J Appl Physiol 31:338-344, 1971

2. Komi PV, Viitasalo JHT, Havu M, Thorstenson H, Sjodin B, Karlson J: Skeletal muscle fibers and muscle enzyme activites in monozygous and dizygous twins of both sexes. Acta Physiol Scand 100:385-392, 1977

3. Rowell LB: Human cardiovascular adjustments to exercise and thermal stress. Physiol Rev 54:75-159, 1974

4. Burke RE, Edgerton VR: Motor unit properties and selective involvement in movement. In, Exercise and Sports Sciences Review. (Wilmore JH, Keogh JF, eds). New York, Academic Press, 1975, Vol 3, p 31

5. Johnson RL, Jr: Oxygen transport. In, Clinical Cardiology. (Willerson JT, Sanders CA, eds). New York, Grune and Stratton, 1977, p 74

6. Saltin B, Henrikson J, Nygaard E, Andersen P: Fiber types and metabolic potentials of skeletal muscles in sedentary man and endurance runners. Ann NY Acad Sci 301:3-29, 1977

7. Holloszy JO, Booth FW: Biochemical adaptations to endurance training in muscle. Ann Rev Physiol 38:273-291, 1976

8. Gollnick PD, Sembrowich WL: Adaptations in human skeletal muscle as a result of training. In, Exercise in Cardiovascular Health and Disease. (Amsterdam EA, Wilmore JH, DeMaria AN, eds). New York, Yorke Medical Books, 1977, p 94

9. Kaiser L: Limiting factors for aerobic muscle performance. Acta Physiol Scand (suppl) 346:1-96, 1970

10. Orlander J, Kiessling KH, Karlson J, Ekblom B: Low intensity training, inactivity, and resumed activity in sedentary men. Acta Physiol Scand 101:351-362, 1977

11. Fagreus L, Karlson J, Linnarson D, Saltin B: Oxygen uptake during maximal work at lowered and raised ambient air pressures. Acta Physiol Scand 87:411-421, 1973

12. Clausen JP: Circulatory adjustments to dynamic exercise and effect of physical training in normal subjects and in patients with coronary artery disease. Prog Cardiovasc Dis 18:459-495, 1975

13. Clausen JP: Effect of physical training on cardio-
    vascular adjustments to exercise in man. Physiol
    Rev 57:779-815, 1977

14. Scheuer J, Tipton CM: Cardiovascular adaptations to
    physical training. Ann Rev Physiol 39:221-251, 1977

15. Saltin B: Central circulation after physical condi-
    tioning in young and middle-aged men. In, Coronary
    Heart Disease and Physical Fitness. Larsen OA,
    Malmborg EO, eds). Munksgaard, Copenhagen, 1971,
    p 26

16. Detry JMR, Rousseau M, Vandenbroucke G, Kusumi F,
    Brasseur LA, Bruce RA: Increased arteriovenous oxy-
    gen difference after physical training in coronary
    disease. Circulation 44:109-118, 1971

17. Detry JMR: Exercise Testing and Training in Coro-
    nary Heart Disease. Baltimore, Williams and Wilkins,
    1973

18. Shephard RJ: Intensity, duration, and frequency of
    exercise as determinants of the response to a train-
    ing regimen. Int Z Angew Physiol 26:272-278, 1968

19. Pollock ML: The quantification of endurance train-
    ing programs. In, Exercise and Sports Sciences
    Reviews. (Wilmore JH, ed). New York, Academic
    Press, 1973, Vol 1, p 188

20. Nordesjo LO: The effect of quantitated training on
    the capacity for short and prolonged work. Acta
    Physiol Scand (suppl) 405:1-54, 1974

21. Kilbom A: Physical training in women. Scand J Clin
    Lab Invest (suppl) 119:1-34, 1971

22. Karvonen MJ, Kentala E, Mustala O: The effects of
    training on heart rate. A longitudinal study. Ann
    Med Exp Fenn 35:307-315, 1957

23. Roskamm H: Optimum patterns of exercise for healthy
    adults. Can Med Assoc J 96:895-900, 1967

24. Kilbom A: Effect on women of physical training
    with low intensities. Scand J Clin Lab Invest
    28:345-352, 1971

25. Siegel W, Blomqvist CG, Mitchell JH: Effects of a
    quantitated physical training program on middle-aged
    sedentary men. Circulation 41:19-29, 1970

26. Saltin B: The interplay between peripheral and cen-
     tral factors in the adaptive response to exercise
     and training. Ann NY Acad Sci 301:224-242, 1977

27. Stone HL: The unanesthetized instrumented animal
     preparation (Symposium on experimental preparations
     to study the effect of training on the cardiovascu-
     lar system). Med Sci Sports 9:253-261, 1977

28. Andrew CM, Guzman CA, Becklake MR: Effect of ath-
     letic training on exercise cardiac output. J Appl
     Physiol 21:603-608, 1966

29. Hanson JS, Tabakin BS, Levy AM, Nedde W: Long-term
     physical training and cardiovascular dynamics in
     middle-aged men. Circulation 38:783-799, 1968

30. Ekblom B: Effect of physical training on oxygen
     transport system in man. Acta Physiol Scand (suppl)
     328:5-45, 1969

31. Saltin B, Blomqvist CG, Mitchell JH, Johnson RL Jr,
     Wildenthal K, Chapman CB: Response to exercise
     after bed rest and after training. Circulation
     (suppl) 7, 38:1-78, 1968

32. Rowell LB: Factors affecting the prediction of the
     maximal oxygen intake from measurements made during
     submaximal work with observations related to factors
     which may limit maximal oxygen intake. PhD Thesis,
     University of Minnesota, 1962

33. Hartley LH, Grimby G, Kilbom A, Nilson WJ, Astrand
     I, Bjure J, Ekblom B, Saltin B: Physical training
     in sedentary middle-aged and older men. Scand J
     Clin Lab Invest 24:335-344, 1969

34. Varnauskas E, Bergman H, Houk P, Bjorntorp P: Hemo-
     dynamic effects of physical training in coronary
     patients. Lancet 2:8-12, 1966

35. Sanne H: Exercise tolerance and physical training
     of non-selected patients after myocardial infarc-
     tion. Acta Med Scand (suppl) 551, 1973

36. Holmgren A, Strandell T: The relationship between
     heart volume, total hemoglobin and physical working
     capacity in former athletes. Acta Med Scand 163:149-
     160, 1959

37. Musshoff K, Reindell H, Klepzig H: Stroke volume,
     arteriovenous differences, cardiac output and physi-
     cal working capacity and their relationship to
     heart volume. Acta Cardiol 14:427-452, 1959

38. Pyorala K, Karvonen MJ, Taskinen P, Takkunen J, Kyronseppa H, Peltokallio P: Cardiovascular studies on former endurance athletes. Am J Cardiol 20:191-205, 1967

39. Saltin B, Grimby G: Physiological analyses of middle-aged and old former athletes. Comparison with still active athletes of the same ages. Circulation 38:1104-1115, 1968

40. Astrand PO, Rodahl K: Textbook of Work Physiology (2nd Edition), New York, McGraw-Hill, 1977

41. Ehsani AA, Hagberg JM, Hickson RC: Rapid changes in left ventricular dimensions and mass in response to physical conditioning and deconditioning. Am J Cardiol 42:52-56, 1978

42. Erikson BO, Lundin A, Saltin B: Cardiopulmonary function in former girl swimmers and the effects of physical training. Scand J Clin Lab Invest 35:135-150, 1975

43. Morganroth J, Baron BJ, Henry WL, Epstein SE: Comparative left ventricular dimensions in trained athletes. Ann Intern Med 82:521-524, 1975

44. Roeske WR, O'Rourke RA, Klein A, Leopold G, Karliner JS: Non-invasive evaluation of ventricular hypertrophy in professional athletes. Circulation 53:286-292, 1975

45. DeMaria AN, Neuman A, Lee G, Fowler W, Mason DT: Alterations in ventricular mass and performance induced by exercise training in man evaluated by echocardiography. Circulation 57:237, 1978

46. Longhurst JC, Kelly AR, Gonyea WJ, Mitchell JH: Left ventricular mass in athletes (abstr). Med Sci Sports 11:82, 1979

47. Rerych SK, Scholz PM, Sabiston DC, Jones RH: Effects of training on left ventricular function in normal subjects: a longitudinal study (abstr). Am J Cardiol 43:1067, 1979

48. Frick MH, Katila M, Sjogren AL: Cardiac function and physical training after myocardial infarction. In, Coronary Heart Disease and Physical Fitness (Larsen OA, Malmborg RO, eds), Copenhagen, Munksgaard, 1971, p 451

49. Wallace AG, Rerych SK, Jones RH, Goodrich JK: Effects of exercise training on ventricular function

in coronary disease (abstr). Circulation 57&58, (suppl) II-97, 1978

50. Wyatt HL, Mitchell JH: Influences of physical conditioning and deconditioning on coronary vasculature of dogs. J Appl Physiol 45:619-625, 1978

51. Holmberg S, Serzysko W, Varnauskas E: Coronary circulation during heavy exercise in control subjects and patients with coronary heart disease. Acta Med Scand 190:465-480, 1971

52. Jorgensen CR, Gobel FL, Taylor HL, Wang Y: Myocardial blood flow and oxygen consumption during exercise. Ann NY Acad Sci 301:213-223, 1977

53. Heaton WH, Marr KC, Capurro NL, Goldstein RE, Epstein JE: Beneficial effect of physical training on blood flow to myocardium perfused by chronic collateral in the exercising dog. Circulation 58: 575-581, 1978

54. Ferguson R, Petitclerc R, Choquette G, Chaniotis L, Gauthier P, Huot P, Allard C, Jankowski L, Campbell L: Effect of physical training on treadmill exercise capacity, collateral circulation and programs of coronary disease. Am J Cardiol 34:764-769, 1974

55. Sim DN, Neill WA: Investigation of the physiological basis for increased exercise threshold for angina pectoris after physical conditioning. J Clin Invest 54:763-770, 1974

56. Scheuer J: The advantages and disadvantages of the isolated perfused working rat heart (Symposium on experimental preparations to study the effect of

    training on the cardiovascular system). Med Sci Sports 9:231-238, 1977

57. Nutter DO, Fuller EO: The role of isolated cardiac muscle preparation in the study of training effects on the heart. Med Sci Sports 9:239-245, 1977

58. Mole PA: Increased contractile potential of papillary muscles from exercise-trained rat hearts. Am J Physiol 234:H421-H425, 1978

59. Wyatt HL, Chuck L, Rabinowitz B, Tyberg JV, Parmley WW: Enhanced cardiac response to catecholamines in physically trained cats. Am J Physiol 234:H608-H613, 1978

60. Green JF: Determinants of systemic blood flow. In, International Review of Physiology, Vol 18. Cardio-vascular Physiology III. (Guyton AC, Young DB, eds). Baltimore, University Park Press, 1979, p 65

61. Robinson FB, Epstein SE, Kahler RL, Braunwald E: Circulatory effects of acute expansion of blood volume. Studies during maximal exercise and at rest. Circ Res 19:26-32, 1966

62. Ekblom B, Wilson G, Astrand PO: Central circulation during exercise after venesection and reinfusion of red blood cells. J Appl Physiol 40:379-383, 1976

63. Bevegard S, Holmgren A, Jonsson B: Circulating studies in well trained athletes at rest and during heavy exercise with special reference to stroke volume and the influence of body position. Acta Physiol Scand 57:26-50, 1963

64. Strandell T: Circulatory studies on healthy old men. Acta Med Scand, (suppl) 414, 1964

65. Mitchell JH, Reardon WC, McClosky DI, Wildenthal K: Possible role of muscle receptors on the cardiovas-cular response to exercise. Ann NY Acad Sci 301: 232-242, 1977

66. Longhurst JC, Mitchell JH: Reflex control of the circulation by afferents from skeletal muscle. In, Cardiovascular Physiology III, Vol 18. (Guyton AC, Young DB, eds). Baltimore, University Park Press, 1979, p 148

67. Bonde-Petersen F, Rowell LB, Murray RG, Blomqvist CG, White R, Karlsson E, Campbell W, Mitchell JH: Role of cardiac output in the pressor responses to graded muscle ischemia in man. J Appl Physiol 45: 574-580, 1978

68. Tipton CM, Matthes RD, Tcheng TK, Dowell RT, Vailas AC: The use of the Langerdorff preparation to study the bradycardia of training. Med Sci Sports 9:220-230, 1977

69. Cooksey JD, Reilly P, Brown S, Bomze H, Cryer PE: Exercise training and plasma catecholamines in patients with ischemic heart disease. Am J Cardiol 42:372-376, 1978

70. Ekstrom J: Choline acetyltransferase in the heart and salivary glands of rats after physical training. Q J Exp Physiol 59:73-80, 1974

71. Lewis SF: Central versus peripheral cardiovascular effects of endurance training with special reference to the mechanisms of bradycardia. PhD Thesis, Stanford University, Stanford, California, 1977

72. Jensen D: Intrinsic Cardiac Rate Regulation. New York, Meredith Corp, 1971

73. Vetrovec GW, Abel PM: Results of exercise conditioning in propranolol and non-propranolol treated patients trained at low heart rates (abstr). Circulation 55&56 (suppl) III:197, 1977

74. Welton DE, Squires WG, Hartung GH, Miller RR: Effects of chronic beta-adrenergic blockade therapy on exercise training in patients with coronary heart disease (abstr). Am J Cardiol 43:399, 1979

75. Lester RM, Wallace AG: Cardiovascular adaptations to beta-adrenergic blockade during physical training (abstr). Circulation 57&58 (suppl) II:140, 1978

76. Tuttle RR, Mills J: Dobutamide: development of a new catecholamine to selectively increase cardiac contractility. Circ Res 36:185-196, 1975

77. Siltovouri A, Tirri R, Harri MNE: Alpha-receptor subsensitivity of isolated atria from rats following physical training or repeated ACTH injections. Acta Physiol Scand 99:457-461, 1977

5

EVALUATION OF MYOCARDIAL PERFUSION AND OXYGEN CONSUMPTION DURING EXERCISE

Francis J. Klocke, M.D.
Avery K. Ellis, M.D.

During exercise the coronary circulation has the usual task of providing an adequate oxygen supply for the heart's metabolic demand. Figure 1 illustrates factors influencing the balance between myocardial O_2 demand and supply. Hemodynamic factors affecting demand have recently been reviewed by Parmley and Tyberg.[1] Of major importance are wall stress, heart rate, and contractile state. Increases in coronary blood flow remain the major mechanism for augmenting O_2 supply, although coronary $A-VO_2$ difference can also increase modestly.

Since myocardial O_2 consumption cannot ordinarily be measured during exercise, a number of investigators have used the product of peak (or mean) systolic blood pressure nd heart rate as an index of O_2 demand. Potential limitations of systolic pressure as an index of wall stress relate to inter- and intraindividual differences in wall thickness and/or ventricular cavity size. Efforts to incorporate contractility into a hemodynamic index of O_2 demand have been of limited value. Potential changes in coronary $A-VO_2$ extraction are ordinarily also neglected.

Direct measurements of myocardial O_2 consumption in man during exercise have been reported by groups from Minnesota[2,4] and Goteborg.[5] The Minnesota group employed nitrous oxide saturation to quantify coronary flow in normal young males studied at two to three levels of exertion using upright bicycle ergometry. The highest levels of exercise achieved corresponded to 85 percent of maximal heart rate and 56 percent of maximal total body oxygen consumption. The $A-VO_2$ difference across the coronary bed increased by 10 to 15 percent, and myocardial O_2 consumption by 300 to 400 percent (assuming usual resting values of this parameter). Indices of O_2

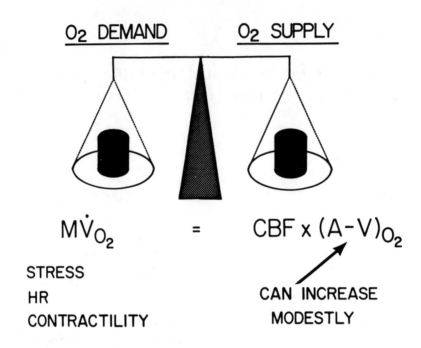

Figure 1:   Evaluation of Myocardial Perfusion

consumption involving the product of systolic pressure and heart rate correlated with CBF (r = 0.87-0.89) myocardial O_2 consumption (r = 0.90) better than tension time index, heart rate, etc. The usefulness of "double product" as an index of myocardial O_2 consumption in groups of healthy, normal individuals was therefore established. However, 95 percent confidence limits for estimates of O_2 consumption from individual values of double product were substantial, i.e., ± 8 ml $O_2/100$ g LV/min (figure 3, reference 4).

In the study of the Goteborg group,[5] myocardial flow was measured from a monoexponential clearance constant derived following bolus injection of Xe^{133} into a coronary artery. Patients were studied supine rather than upright, using an electrically braked bicycle ergometer. The double product of systolic pressure and heart rate was in the same range as in the Minnesota studies and was again reported to be a useful index of myocardial O_2 uptake in control subjects. The slope of the regression line calculated for these subjects is less than the slope of the similar line for the entire Minnesota group of normal individuals[4] [MVO_2 = 0.097 DP 0.62, r = 0.89 vs. MVO_2 = 0.16 DP - 3.9, r^2 = 0.85]. It should be noted that 95 percent confidence limits for prediction of O_2 uptake from individual measurements of double product again vary widely.

Similar data reported by the Goteborg group for patients with coronary artery disease seem difficult to interpret in light of the potential limitations of the Xe^{133} technique in this setting.[6]

The Minnesota group repeated studies in normal male volunteers before and after beta blockade, again using upright bicycle exercise.[4] Their findings emphasize that relative metabolic loads for the whole body and heart are determined separately, and do not necessarily change in parallel with a given intervention. Following systemic beta blockade with propranolol, a significantly higher workload was required to achieve a heart rate of 120 beats/min, although double product and myocardial O_2 consumption were the same at the two workloads. Similarly, when exercise to a given workload was repeated after propranolol, the workload was achieved at significantly lower values of double product and myocardial O_2 consumption. The rate pressure product continued to correlate well with myocardial O_2 consumption, despite the reduction in contractility produced by this agent. The continued correlation may, at least in part, have reflected "cancelling" effects of directionally opposite influences on O_2 consumption, e.g., reduced contractility secondary to propranolol vs. increased wall stress secondary to a larger heart size during exercise. Also noteworthy was an 18 percent greater coronary A-V O_2 extraction at the same level of double product (16.1 ml O_2/100 ml with propranolol vs. 13.8 ml O_2/100 ml prior to propranolol).

When patients with ischemic heart disease caused by coronary atherosclerosis are exercised, the situation is more complex. Regional variations in myocardial perfusion and/or performance may occur at rest[7,8] and certainly do so during exercise. Studies in experimental animals with partial coronary artery obstruction have demonstrated exercise-related transmural redistribution of flow, with relative subendocardial underperfusion.[9] Dramatic changes in regional performance, sometimes leading to cardiac arrest, have also been documented during exercise in chronically instrumented animals with restricted coronary inflow.[10] Effects of collateral circulation remain difficult to sort out, in view of varying reports in different species and experimental preparations.[11,16] At present, the evaluation of regional myocardial performance seems the best index of changes in the local balance between myocardial O_2 supply and demand in man. Noninvasive approaches for making this evaluation have progressed rapidly and appear promising for sequential evaluation of individual patients during training.

79

Physical training may have several beneficial effects on the coronary circulation. It is well-established that myocardial O_2 requirements are less for any given level of exercise in a trained individual. The diminished heart rate is an important factor in this response, while effects of hypertrophy and/or cavity dilation[17] are more difficult to sort out. In addition to reducing O_2 demand, the slower heart rate allows a greater duration of diastolic coronary perfusion. Several studies suggest that myocardial capillary density may be increased by training.[18,20] Reported effects of training on collateral perfusion vary, a positive effect being noted in fox hounds[15] and no effect in miniature swine.[16] Wyatt and colleagues[21] have suggested that training augments the effects of catecholamines on myocardial contractility without a change in intrinsic contractile function. Little information is available about the effects of training on local myocardial tissue pressure, although this parameter might influence local perfusion independently of metabolically-induced dilation of resistance vessels.

An additional factor influencing coronary perfusion and the calculation of coronary vascular resistance which has been appreciated only recently is illustrated in figures 2 and 3. Figure 2 schematically represents traditional concepts of pressure-flow relations within the coronary vascular bed. The solid black line depicts the relationship between flow and pressure over a wide range of these values. The range of pressure over which flow remains relatively constant--the so-called "autoregulatory" range--lies between the bounds of maximum vasodilation and maximum vasoconstriction. The black dot represents a typical operating point within this autoregulatory range. Vascular resistance calculated for this point usually employs the hydraulic equivalent of Ohm's Law, R = P/Q. The choice of P has varied, sometimes being taken as the difference between inflow and right atrial pressures, and sometimes as inflow pressure alone. During the past few years attention has focused increasingly on the difference between inflow and left ventricular (or atrial) diastolic pressures since local tissue pressure may limit flow even during diastole. Previous studies of autoregulation suggest that the minimum pressure required for any flow during maximum vasodilation is slightly higher than either right or left atrial pressures.[22,24] Thus, the proper choice of driving pressure is at issue. Overestimates of driving pressure will, of course, lead to overestimates of coronary vascular resistance.

Figure 3 summarizes recently obtained data which indicate that the magnitude of this problem is greater than previously suspected.[24] When instantaneous pressure-flow

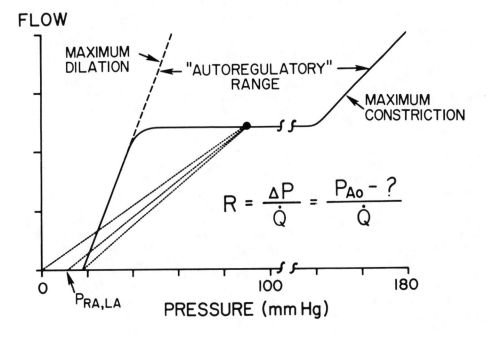

FLOW

MAXIMUM
DILATION

"AUTOREGULATORY"
RANGE

MAXIMUM
CONSTRICTION

$$R = \frac{\Delta P}{\dot{Q}} = \frac{P_{Ao} - ?}{\dot{Q}}$$

0   $P_{RA,LA}$ 100   180

PRESSURE (mm Hg)

Figure 2:   Evaluation of Myocardial Perfusion

Actual Diastolic Pressure – Flow Relation

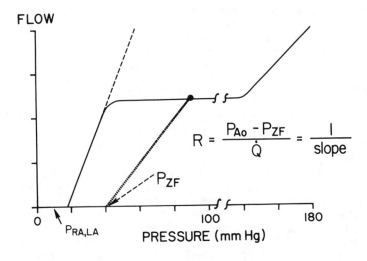

FLOW

$$R = \frac{P_{Ao} - P_{ZF}}{\dot{Q}} = \frac{1}{slope}$$

P_{ZF}

0   $P_{RA,LA}$ 100   180

PRESSURE (mm Hg)

Figure 3:   Evaluation of Myocardial Perfusion

81

relationships were quantitated during single long diastoles in open-chest dogs, flow was consistently a linear function of inflow pressure. The reciprocal of the pressure-flow line provided a direct measure of coronary vascular resistance, and the pressure-axis intercept an estimate of the minimum inflow pressure required for any diastolic perfusion. The latter, termed zero flow pressure (P_{ZF}), was 3 to 5 times greater than mean left or right atrial pressure under control conditions, averaging 32 ± 3.1 (SEM) mm Hg.

This finding is consistent with the recent work of Bellamy[25] suggesting that forces opposing diastolic flow in the immediate vicinity of intramyocardial vascular channels are higher than previously considered. The minimum pressure required for any diastolic flow in Bellamy's studies was 40 mm Hg under basal conditions, but decreased following total inflow occlusion or maximum pharmacologic vasodilation. P_{ZF} has now also been shown to vary during modest changes in coronary pressure and flow (which traditionally would have been attributed entirely to changes in coronary resistance).[24] Thus, P_{ZF} normally exerts a quantitatively important back pressure to flow, and coronary vascular resistance can be overestimated importantly if it is ignored. Options for adjusting coronary flow are more complex than suggested by traditional concepts of autoregulation, since they include changes in position as well as slope of the diastolic pressure-flow relationship. While it is clear that coronary vascular resistance decreases importantly during exercise, concomitant changes in P_{ZF} are difficult to predict, particularly in the presence of coronary artery disease.

In summary, hemodynamic "double product" indices of myocardial O_2 requirements are quite useful in evaluating groups of normal subjects, although there is significant scatter among individual values. The indices also appear useful in the presence of beta blockade, emphasizing that relative metabolic loads for the heart and body need not change similarly with a given intervention.

The usefulness of all hemodynamic indices is more tenuous when regional and/or transmural variations in myocardial perfusion and performance are likely. Such is clearly the case in ischemic heart disease caused by coronary atherosclerosis. Physical training has several potentially beneficial effects on the coronary circulation. It is well-established that myocardial O_2 requirements are less for any given level of exercise in the trained individual. Traditional concepts relating to driving pressure within the coronary bed and the calculation of coronary vascular resistance need to be reexamined in light of recent information about the minimum inflow pressure required for any diastolic perfusion.

The latter is of substantial magnitude, and varies appreciably in response to different hemodynamic and pharmacologic interventions.

Additional fundamental information about myocardial perfusion and performance during exercise and training is clearly needed. Detailed information of this type will almost certainly have to be obtained in experimental animals subjected to extensive chronic instrumentation. Such studies will need to include observations with and without simulation of coronary stenosis. Even with simulation of local stenosis, extrapolation of findings to man will require considerable caution, since human coronary artery atherosclerosis commonly has an appreciable longitudinal extent.[26,28] Traditional hemodynamic indices will continue to be useful in evaluating overall cardiac performance in man, but noninvasive evaluation of regional myocardial performance seems likely to provide the most sensitive index of changes in the local balance between demand and supply.

References

1. Parmley WW, Tyberg JV: Determination of myocardial oxygen demand. In, Progress in Cardiology, Vol 5 (Yu PN, Goodwin JF, eds). Philadelphia, Lea and Febiger, 1976, p 19

2. Jorgensen CR, Kitamura K, Gobel FL, Taylor HL, Wang Y: Long-term precision of the N_2O method for coronary flow during heavy upright exercise. J Appl Physiol 30:338-344, 1971

3. Kitamura K, Jorgensen CR, Gobel FL, Taylor HL, Wang Y: Hemodynamic correlates of myocardial oxygen consumption during upright exercise. J Appl Physiol 32:516-522, 1972

4. Jorgensen CR, Wang K, Wang Y, Gobel FL, Nelson RR, Taylor H: Effect of propranolol on myocardial oxygen consumption and its hemodynamic correlates during upright exercise. Circulation 48:1173-1182, 1973

5. Holmberg S, Serzysko W, Varnauskas E: Coronary circulation during heavy exercise in control subjects and patients with coronary heart disease. Acta Med Scand 190:465-480, 1971

6. Klocke FJ: Coronary blood flow in man. Prog Cardiovasc Dis 19:117116, 1976

7. Klocke FJ, Greene DG, Bunnell IL, Roberts DL, Dashkoff N, Arani DT: Relationship between degree of stenosis and reductions in regional myocardial blood flow in coronary artery disease. Clin Res 502A, 1979

8. St John Sutton MG, Frye RL, Smith HC, Chesbro JH, Ritman EL: Relation between left coronary artery stenosis and regional left ventricular function. Circulation 58:491-497, 1978

9. Ball RM, Bache RJ: Distribution of myocardial blood flow in the exercising dog with restricted coronary artery inflow. Circ Res 38:60-66, 1976

10. Tomoike H, Franklin D, McKown D, Kemper WS, Guberek M, Ross J Jr: Regional myocardial dysfunction and hemodynamic abnormalities during strenuous exercise in dogs with limited coronary flow. Circ Res 42: 487-496, 1978

11. Gregg DE: The natural history of coronary collateral development. Circ Res 35:335-344, 1974

12. Schaper W, Flameng W, Winkler B, Wusten B, Turschmann W, Neugebauer G, Carl M, Psayk S: Quantification of collateral resistance in acute and choronic experimental coronary occlusion in the dog. Circ Res 39:371377, 1976

13. Lambert PR, Hess DS, Bache RJ: Effect of exercise on perfusion of collateral-dependent myocardium in dogs with chronic coronary artery occlusion. J Clin Invest 59:1-7, 1977

14. Cohen MV, Yipintsoi T, Malhotra A, Scheuer J: Effect of exercise on coronary collateral function. Am J Cardiol 39:262, 1977

15. Heaton WH, Marr KC, Capurro NL, Goldstein RE, Epstein SE: Beneficial effect of physical training on blood flow to myocardium perfused by chronic collaterals in the exercising dog. Circulation 57:575-581, 1978

16. Sanders M, White FC, Peterson TM, Bloor CM: Effects of endurance exercise on coronary collateral blood flow in miniature swine. Am J Physiol 234:H614-H619, 1978

17. Wyatt HL, Mitchell JH: Influences of physical training on the heart of dogs. Circ Res 35:883-889, 1974

18. Wyatt HL, Mitchell JH: Influences of physical conditioning and deconditioning upon the coronary vasculature of dogs. Am J Cardiol 39:262, 1977

19. McElroy CL, Gissen SA, Fishbein MC: Exercise-induced reduction in myocardial infarct size after coronary artery occlusion in the rat. Circulation 57:958-962, 1978

20. Leon AS, Bloor CM: Effects of exercise and its cessation on the heart and its blood supply. J Appl Physiol 24:485-490, 1968

21. Wyatt HL, Chuck L, Rabinowitz B, Tyberg JV, Parmley WW: Enhanced cardiac response to catecholamines in physically trained cats. Am J Physiol 234:H608-H613, 1978

22. Mosher P, Ross J, McFate PA, Shaw RF: Control of coronary blood flow by an autoregulatory mechanism. Circ Res 14:250-259, 1964

23. Ellis AK, Klocke FJ: Effects of preload on the transmural distribution of perfusion and pressure-flow relationships in the canine coronary vascular bed. Submitted for publication.

24. Ellis AK, Klocke FJ: Changes in coronary perfusion with or without changes in coronary vascular resistance: complexities of driving pressure and autoregulation. Submitted for publication.

25. Bellamy RF: Diastolic coronary artery pressure-flow relations in the dog. Circ Res 43:92-101, 1978

26. Jones AA, Roberts WC: Quantitation of coronary artery narrowing in sudden coronary death. Circulation 58:II133, (No. 516), 1978

27. Arnett EN, Isner JM, Redwood DR, Kent K, Baker WP, Ackerstein H, Roberts WC: Underestimation by angiography of critical coronary arterial narrowing in life: comparison with degree of narrowing assessed by quantitative histological examination at necropsy. Am J Cardiol 43:343, 1979

28. Varmani R, Roberts WC: Quantitation of coronary artery narrowing in clinically-isolated angina pectoris. Am J Cardiol 43:343, 1979

6

INFLUENCE OF HABITUAL PHYSICAL ACTIVITY ON BLOOD LIPIDS AND LIPOPROTEINS

William L. Haskell, Ph.D.

The recent resurgence of interest in the relationship between the level of habitual physical activity and the concentration of blood lipids or lipoproteins was precipitated by the recognition of low levels of plasma high density lipoprotein-cholesterol (HDL-C) as a risk factor for atherosclerotic vascular disease. Low concentrations of HDL-C are associated with increased risk for the clinical manifestations of coronary heart disease, peripheral vascular disease and stroke and the acceleration of coronary atherosclerosis as determined by arteriography. This inverse relationship between HDL-C concentration and various manifestations of atherosclerotic vascular disease generally appears to be independent of other established risk factors, including other blood lipids or lipoproteins.

The present paper reviews our current state of knowledge regarding the influence of habitual physical activity on blood lipid and lipoprotein levels, with special emphasis given to studies of HDL-C in man. The blood lipids of total cholesterol and triglycerides will be considered first, then the lipoproteins, very low density lipoprotein-cholesterol (VLDL-C), low density lipoprotein-cholesterol (LDL-C), and HDL-C. Several reviews regarding exercise and lipid metabolism were published recently.[1,2]

Total Cholesterol

Cross-sectional and longitudinal studies of total blood cholesterol concentration (plasma or serum) generally indicate that more physically active individuals

tend to have similar or somewhat lower total cholesterol
levels than their inactive counterparts.[3-5] In studies
reporting lower levels in more active adults, usually
the magnitude of this difference is within 6 percent
when values are adjusted for variations in adiposity.
When a reduction in total cholesterol is reported as a
result of exercise training, this decrease frequently
is associated with a decrease in body weight, and in
some cases this decrease in weight is of a magnitude
greater than can be accounted for by the increase in
caloric expenditure, suggesting some change in dietary
intake.

Several reports indicate that significantly lower
total cholesterol levels (compared to sedentary controls)
are associated with vigorous activity, for instance in
cross-country runners and skiers;[6] in middle-aged male
and female long distance runners.[7] On the other hand,
many studies have failed to show significant differences
between active groups and sedentary controls: for instance, in male marathon runners aged 24 to 43;[8] in
English male civil servants aged 40 to 64 who reported
vigorous leisure time activity;[9] in Norwegian male
cross-country skiers aged 16 to 74;[10] in Finnish male
runners and skiers aged 35 to 68;[11] and in Finnish lumberjacks.[12] A study by Montoye et al.[13] on 1060 males
and 119 females from the Tecumseh Community Health
Study reported no relationship between maximal oxygen
uptake (a measure of physical fitness) and plasma total
cholesterol concentration, when the effects of age,
weight and adiposity were removed. Similar results have
been observed in data from the collaborative Lipid Research Clinics prevalence study.[14]

As might be predicted from the results of these cross-
sectional observations, longitudinal studies have provided no clear consensus on the question of exercise in
relation to plasma total cholesterol concentration. In
several studies on normal subjects,[4,15,16] a significant
decrease in total cholesterol has accompanied exercise
training. Campbell[17] noted that vigorous, dynamic
sports, in particular cross-country running and tennis,
resulted in significant decreases in total cholesterol
in young male students, whereas relatively static sports,
such as wrestling and weight training, did not. Melish
et al.[18] found a significant reduction in total cholesterol following a 6-month exercise program in a group of
Type II hyperlipoproteinemic men. Considerable reductions in plasma total cholesterol have been reported in
circumstances where caloric restriction and significant
weight loss accompanied the exercise.[19] A report in
abstract by Weltman et al.[20] suggests that an exercise
program alone is equally as effective as exercise plus
diet (presumably a weight-loss diet) in bringing about
reduction of plasma total cholesterol concentration.

On the other hand, a number of authors have reported no significant change in total cholesterol concentration during a variety of short-term and longer-term exercise programs.[3,8,21,23] Several of these studies showed considerable significance was not reached. In three studies[24-26] Type IV men (with elevated triglycerides and VLDL) showed a reduction of triglyceride level with exercise, but cholesterol concentration change was not significant.

Triglycerides

In contrast to total cholesterol, exercise does appear to have a unique or independent effect on plasma triglycerides. Performance of large muscle dynamic exercise frequently results in a reduction in the plasma triglyceride (TG) levels of hypertriglyceridemic adults. This reduction appears to have both acute and chronic components: following endurance type exercise, triglyceride concentration is temporarily lowered in many hypertriglyceridemic subjects[24,25] and more physically active individuals generally have lower TG levels than less active men or women of a similar age.[5] The lower TG levels in the more active adults cannot be fully accounted for by their lower body mass index (BMI) or dietary intake. Individuals with low TG levels usually do not demonstrate much further lowering with exercise training.

Comparison of very active cross-country skiers and runners with sedentary adults supports an association between lower TG levels and an elevation in lipoprotein lipase concentrations in adipose and/or skeletal muscle tissue.[27] These data have not been adjusted for other characteristics (BMI, diet, etc.) nor have any data from well-controlled training studies been reported. An increase in lipoprotein lipase, however, has been reported as a result of exercise training in rats.[28]

Bjorntorp et al.[6] reported significantly lower triglyceride concentrations for 15 physically well-trained men aged 52 to 56, compared with 45 sedentary control men. Hurter et al.[8] similarly found lower plasma triglyceride levels in younger male long-distance runners compared to sedentary men. Using standardized assays, Wood et al.[5] examined 41 male and 43 female long-distance runners, randomly selected from three northern California towns, while Martin et al.[7] reported on 20 young elite male runners and sedentary controls. Lehtonen and Viikari[11] measured lower triglycerides in 23 men aged 35 to 68 who were running or skiing 83 km per week in comparison with 15 healthy but inactive men aged 33 to 58. The same authors[12] also found lower plasma triglyceride levels in 12 Finnish lumberjacks compared with levels in 15 electricians; this study suggests that vigorous physical activity at work, as well as vigorous leisure time activity, results in relatively low plasma triglyceride concentrations.

These and other studies are consistent in their findings of low mean triglyceride levels in physically very active groups. It is noteworthy that the spread of values (as indicated by standard deviations) is also consistently lower in the active groups. Measurements of VLDL-cholesterol in male and female long-distance runners have confirmed that the triglyceride-rich VLDL is indeed at a very low level in these very active individuals.[5]

The acute effects of vigorous exercise on plasma triglycerides have been studied by several investigators. Carlson and Mossfeldt[21] found a significant mean decrease in triglycerides from 108 to 69 mg/100 ml in male participants in an 85 km ski race. Carlson and Froberg[19] reported on a group of 12 men who walked 50 km per day for 10 days with very little caloric intake. Plasma triglyceride fell by more than 50 percent after 3 days, and then rose slightly over the next 7 exercising days. Participants lost a considerable amount of weight during the walk. Oscai et al.[24] exercised seven hypertriglyceridemic, middle-aged men during 4 successive days by having them run 3 to 4 miles in 40 minutes each day. Mean plasma triglyceride at baseline was 235 mg/100 ml, while levels after successive days of exercise were 173, 136, 119, and 104 mg/100 ml. Most of these differences were significant. Hunter et al.[8] measured triglycerides in 14 trained male athletes before and after a marathon race and found a small but insignificant increase. A variable degree of hemoconcentration probably occurs in these acute exercise studies, tending to increase concentrations of all lipoproteins temporarily.

Several investigators have examined triglyceride changes following exercise in subjects who were initially hyperlipoproteinemic. Holloszy et al.[3] studied 15 professional men, aged 35 to 55, whose initially high mean triglyceride (208 mg/100 ml) fell to a mean of 125 mg/100 ml during the course of a 6-month program of distance running and calisthenics. Oscai et al.[24] found a progressive decrease in triglycerides to normal levels among seven hypertriglyceridemic males during 4 days of exercise. Gyntelberg et al.[25] found a significant decrease in mean plasma triglyceride in five Type IV subjects who exercised by walking for 30 minutes on a treadmill for 4 days. This decrease occurred whether or not the increased caloric expenditure was compensated for by increased food intake. Lampman et al.[26] examined the effect of 10 weeks of high intensity physical training on 23 middle-aged men with Type IV hyperlipoproteinemia and report a significant decrease in both plasma triglycerides and insulin. Melish et al.[18] reported (abstract) on 29 men with Type II hyperlipoproteinemia (elevated LDL); 18 exercised for 6 months while 11 acted as sedentary controls.

Lastly, some observations have been made in subjects with proven CHD. For instance, Erkelens et al.[29] reported (abstract) that 18 survivors of myocardial infarction who exercised moderately for 3 months showed an unchanged triglyceride concentration.

Cholesterol Composition of Specific Lipoproteins

A number of preliminary studies have included comparisons of physical activity status to one or more of the major specific lipoprotein classes, usually by assay of the cholesterol (esterified plus unesterified) content of the separated HDL, LDL, and VLDL fractions. The results of these studies so far have been somewhat inconsistent with regard to changes in the HDL-C, LDL-C, and VLDL-C: a few studies reported no change while others showed differential increases or decreases in one or more of these lipoproteins.

General Review

VLDL-cholesterol

As with plasma triglycerides, VLDL cholesterol generally is lower in more active adults (but it has only been calculated from triglyceride concentration and not directly measured in most studies). Elite runners or skiers have much lower VLDL-C values than nonathletes[5,11] while more active individuals in the general public have slightly lower VLDL-C than sedentary adults when data are adjusted for adiposity, smoking, and alcohol use.[14]

LDL-cholesterol

Athlete vs. nonathlete studies,[5] cross-sectional studies of the general population,[14] and exercise training studies[23] all indicate that physical activity is, at most, only slightly associated with lower LDL-cholesterol levels. Athletes tend to have modest, but significantly lower, LDL-C than nonathletes,[5] but no such difference is usually observed in the general population when classified according to on-the-job or leisure activity.[14] A significant variation from these findings is a preliminary report that exercise training by Type IIa hyperlipoproteinemic subjects results in a 14 percent decrease in LDL-C (201 to 173 mgs/dl) which was significantly correlated (r = .54) with a decrease in adiposity.[18] A summary of the LDL-C values for endurance athletes vs. nonathletes is provided in table 1.

Table 1: LDL-C Values in Endurance Athletes and Nonathletes

Study	Sex	Nonathlete	Endurance Athlete	%
Wood (5)	Male	139	125	-10
	Female	124	113	- 9
Martin (7)	Male	124	108	-13
Nikkila (27)	Male	128	139	+ 9
	Female	108	116	+ 7
Dale (34)	Female	76	79	+ 4
Lehtonen (12) (lumberjacks vs. electricians)	Male	130	138	+ 6

Mean value in mg/100 ml.

$p > 0.05$.

HDL-cholesterol

Once the rationale for a potential protective effect of HDL-C was presented by Miller and Miller in 1975,[30] data relating increased physical activity to higher values of HDL-C were uncovered. The initial data demonstrating this relationship were from comparisons of endurance athletes vs. nonathletes.[5,10,11] Such studies reported HDL-C values 10 to 40 percent higher for the more active men and women. Data in these reports were not adjusted for other factors such as adiposity, cigarette smoking, or alcohol use--all of which may alter HDL-C concentration. Data from HDL-C cross-sectional studies of athletes and nonathletes are included in table 2.

Table 2: LDL-C Values in Endurance Athletes and Nonathletes

Study	Sex	Nonathlete	Endurance Athlete	%
Wood (5)	Male	43	64	+44*
	Female	56	75	+34*
Martin (7)	Male	49	56	+14*
Enger (10)	Male	55	61	+11*
Lehtonen (11)	Male	55	69	+25*
Nikkila (27)	Male	47	66	+40*
	Female	43	64	+49
Dale (34)	Female	68	86	+26*
Hartung (33)	Male	44	65	+48*

Mean values in mg/100 ml.

*$p < 0.05$.

Cross-sectional studies of the general population have demonstrated an association between self-report of activity and HDL-C. These differences tend to be substantially less than for the comparison of endurance athletes vs. nonathletes with the differences, as demonstrated in table 3, generally being in the range of 5 to 10 percent.[14,31]

Specific Studies

One of the first observations of the association of the vigorously active lifestyle with plasma HDL concentration was that of Carlson and Mossfeldt in 1964;[21] male Swedish skiers showed higher mean HDL-cholesterol levels than had been reported for the general male population.[32] Our group at Stanford conducted several cross-sectional studies, in middle-aged male and female runners[5] and in young, elite long-distance runners,[7] each in comparison with a randomly selected control group of appropriate age and sex. Comparisons were made between groups of dedicated long-distance runners and

Table 3: HDL-C Values in Active vs. Inactive Adults

Study	Sex	Inactive Adults	Active Adults	%
LRC (14)	Male	...	44.0	+6.2
	Female	53.2	56.1	+5.5
Williams (31)	Male	53.7	57.4	+6.9
Lehtonen (11)	Male	55	75	+36

Mean values in mg/100 ml.

age-sex-matched control groups, without any attempt to adjust for factors such as adiposity and smoking habits. From these crude comparisons it was clear that the active groups, in each case, exhibited significantly higher HDL-cholesterol concentrations.

Mean plasma HDL-cholesterol in a group of 220 male Norwegian skiers was significantly higher than that of several control groups of relatively sedentary Norwegian men.[10]. Twenty-three male Finnish runners and skiers (mean age 44) had an HDL-cholesterol that was significantly higher than that of an inactive control group of similar age, according to Lehtonen and Viikari.[11]. These same authors[12] also reported recently that FInnish lumberjacks have significantly higher HDL-cholesterol levels than relatively sedentary electricians of similar age (75 vs. 55 mg/100 ml). This is of interest, since Finnish lumberjacks have often been cited as a group that is not proteched against CHD (they have a high rate) even though they have a very high level of occupational activity, because they ear a particularly atherogenic diet. This study indicates that they do have a high-plasma HDL-cholesterol level, as one might anticipate; but surprisingly, their reported mean total cholesterol (224 mg/100 ml) and calculated LDL-cholesterol (138 mg/100 ml) were not particularly high by U.S. standards.

In a study reported in abstract by Hartung et al.,[33] a group of 59 male marathon runners and a second group of 85 male joggers had significicntly higher plasma HDL-cholesterol levels than a sedentary control group (65 vs. 58 vs. 44 mg/100 ml, respectively). Thus, the joggers exhibited increased HDL-cholesterol levels even though their mean jogging distance was no more than 11

miles/week. The study also failed to show any significant relationship of dietary intake to HDL mevel for men
in these different activity classificantions. Also, recent data from the Lipid Research Clinics prevalence
survey indicate this relationship is largely independent
of differences in body mass index, cigarette smoking,
and alcohol use--more so for men than for women.[14]

Carlson and Mossfeldt in 1964[21] reported on men before
and after participation in an 85-km ski race and showed a
slight but nonsignificant decrease in LDL-cholesterol.
During the course of the 500-km, 10-day walk reported by
Carlson and Frober,[19], the participants showed a large
and continuous decrease in LDL-cholesterol (129 mg/100
ml at baseline reduced to 61 mg/100 ml at the 10th day)
and an increase in HDL-cholesterol that was significant
at the 6th day of the walk (61 mg/100 ml increased to 70
mg/100 ml). Participants experienced considerable weight
loss during the walk. The 39 male subjects (ages 18 to
59) in Altedreuse and Wilmore's training study [16] showed
a significant increase in the mean proportion of alpha-
lipoprotein (HDL) in total lipoprotein after 10 weeks.
The proportions if LDL and VLDL in total lipoprotein
each decreased significantly. Although absolute concentrations of lipoprotein fractions were not determined in
this study, it was one of the first to show a significant
redistribution of plasma lipoproteins in an apparently
desirable direction in a group of initially rather sedentary men followed for only 10 weeks on a not unduly
demanding exercise program (an average of only 5 miles
per week was run at an average speed of 7.5 miles per
hour). The mean weight loss reported was only 2 kilo-
grams.

Lopez et al.[4] studied 13 young male medical students
who underwent an exercise program (jogging, cycling,
calisthenics) of four daily 30-minute sessions per week
for 7 weeks. The mean concentration of alpha lipoprotein
(HDL) increased significantly. Beta lipoprotein (LDL),
and also LDL-cholesterol both decreased significantly,
in agreement with the proportional changes found by
Altekreuse and Wilmore.

The remaining reports of which we are aware, describ-
ing recent longitudinal work in the exercise-plasma lipoprotein area, are at present in abstract form. Leon et
al.[35] observed a significant increase in HDL-cholesterol
in six obese young college men who exercised for 1.5
hours/day for 16 weeks (3 percent loss of body fat).
Ratcliff et al.[23] studied 14 previously untrained middle-
aged firefighters who exercised three times per week for
20 weeks, while 14 others acted as sedentary controls.
The only significant change in lipoprotein cholesterol
levels was an increase in HDL-cholesterol (42 to 50 mg/
100 ml) in exercisers. The percent of body mass as fat

decreased significantly in the exercise group compared to the controls.

Weltman et al.[20] looked at the effects of either 10 weeks of exercise or 10 weeks of exercise plus a weight-loss diet in groups of middle-aged sedentary men and women, versus an untreated control group. There was a significant decrease in total cholesterol and LDL-cholesterol, and a decrease in the LDL-cholesterol/HDL-cholesterol ratio, in the exercising groups whether or not the exercise was accompanied by a weight-loss diet. Melish et al.[18] worked with men (aged 35 to 58) with Type II hyperlipoproteinemia, who were already being treated (by diet only) for their elevated plasma LDL-cholesterol. Eighteen were assigned to an exercise group for 6 months and 11 to a sedentary control group. The exercisers showed significant decrease in total cholesterol and LDL-cholesterol, but no change in HDL-cholesterol. Total body weight did not change in the exercisers, but estimated body fat mass fell from 22.5 to 20.0 percent.

Erkelens et al.[29] reported on 18 survivors of myocardial infarction who underwent a 3-month exercise training program. Compared to the untrained state, mean HDL-cholesterol increased significantly after only one week on the exercise program (35 to 40 mg/1-0 ml) and remained significantly elevated after 3 months of training. There was no significant change in plasma total cholesterol or triglycerides; the LDL-cholesterol level was not reported. The differences in the results of these early training studies cannot be explained using the limited data available, but may be the result of variations in the characteristics of subjects, exercise training programs, measurement procedures or control group selection.

In an attempt to further characterize the HDL elevation that frequently appears among very active runners, we and our coworkers examined a subset of men and women runners using the analytical ultracentrifuge for quantitation of HDL subfractions (HDL_2 and HDL_3) and radial immunodiffusion for assay of apolipoproteins A-I and A-II.[35] Seven male runners (aged 42 to 58) and 6 premenopausal female runners not on hormones (aged 34 to 46) were compared to randomly selected control groups of similar age believed to be representative of the U.S. adult population (table 4). Preliminary conclusions from this small study are as follows: the elevated plasma HDL-cholesterol concentration characteristic of runners (males and females) represents an increased total mass of the HDL fraction. This increase is predominantly in the less-dense, larger particle size HDL_2 subfraction, and is accompanied by an elevation of plasma apolipoprotein A-I but not of apolipoprotein A-II. Thus, it

Table 4: Concentration of HDL Subfractions (HDL_2 and HDL_3), HDL Cholesterol and Apolipoproteins A-I and A-II in Long-Distance Runners and Randomly Selected Controls Aged 30-59[21]

	Runners		Random Controls	
	Males (n=7)	Females (n=6)	Males (n=38)	Females (n=20)
HDL_2	119 $\pm$ 47*	281 $\pm$ 79*	53 $\pm$ 44	122 $\pm$ 85
HDL_3	259 $\pm$ 22†	220 $\pm$ 38†	227 $\pm$ 45	220 $\pm$ 28
Apo-A-I	163 $\pm$ 14*	176 $\pm$ 26*	120 $\pm$ 20	130 $\pm$ 22
Apo-A-II	30 $\pm$ 1†	30 $\pm$ 2†	33 $\pm$ 5	34 $\pm$ 5
HDL Cholesterol	70 $\pm$ 10	85 $\pm$ 27	---	---

Mean $\pm$ SD (mg/dl).

*Mean for runners is significantly different (p<0.05) from control.

†No significant difference between means for runners and controls.

appears that both the protein and lipid mass of HDL-C is higher in very active adults.

Potential Biochemical Mechanisms

The precise mechanisms whereby increased physical activity level might lead to altered concentrations of plasma lipoproteins are not known. However, preliminary evidence does exist for several possibilities. Plasma VLDL concentration is inversely correlated with HDL-cholesterol concentration with very active groups showing remarkably low plasma triglyceride levels. Male long-distance runners have been shown recently to have higher levels of muscle and adipose tissue lipoprotein lipase activity than sedentary controls, and wholebody lipoprotein lipase activity was estimated at 2.3 times higher in the runners. Serum HDL-cholesterol level and lipoprotein lipase activity of adipose tissue correlated highly.[37] It is quite probable that increased physical activity leads to increased muscle and adipose tissue lipoprotein lipase activity which in turn leads to lowered plasma triglyceride concentration and ultimately to increased HDL concentration.

The enzyme LCAT (lecithin-cholesterol acyltransferase), which may be involved in the transfer of unesterified cholesterol from cells to "nascent" HDL, has been reported to have increased activity in exercising rats[38] and humans.[4] The predominant apolipoprotein of HDL, apo-A-I, which is increased in runners compared to controls (table 4) is an essential activator of the LCAT reaction. HDL-cholesterol (unesterified) has been shown recently to be the preferred source of cholesterol (as compared with LDL-cholesterol) for incorporation into human biliary cholesterol[39] and bile acids.[40] In the near future these fragments probably will be put together to reveal the entire spectrum of events among the lipoproteins that ensues when the sedentary individual begins to exercise.

Conclusions

1. Total cholesterol and LDL-C generally vary little with exercise habits.

2. TG and VLDL-C levels are lower and HDL-C levels higher in physically active adults.

3. Higher plasma HDL-C is associated with both job and leisure activity.

4. A dose response effect appears to exist for exercise vs. TG and HDL-C.

5. While TG may be lowered acutely by exercise, HDL-C shows no immediate response to exercise.

6. Some, but not all, HDL-C elevation in the physically active may be due to adiposity, smoking, and alcohol intake differences.

7. Specific lipid (HDL_2) and protein (apo-A-I) portions of HDL appear to be elevated in runners.

8. Increases in lipoprotein lipase activity in the muscle or adipose tissue of very active people may be important in decreasing TG and increasing HDL-C, and thus favorably altering CHD risk.

Recommendations for Research

Appropriately designed and implemented studies are needed to answer the following questions:

1. Will an increase in habitual physical activity by
    sedentary individuals have a significant elevating
    effect on HDL-C (thus lowering the total choles-
    terol/HDL-C ratio) independent of changes in
    adiposity or dietary intake?

2. If an exercise increases HDL-C, what individuals
    (as defined by their lipid or lipoprotein profile)
    will benefit, and can these individuals be readily
    identified?

3. What are the characteristics of physical activity
    (type, intensity, duration, amount) that most
    likely will produce a favorable change in the
    lipoprotein profile? Does some type of threshold
    exist?

4. What is the sequence of biochemical changes re-
    sponsible for any significant lipoprotein changes
    occurring as a result of exercise training? Are
    there age or sex related differences in these
    effects?
5. What changes does progressive exercise training
    produce in specific subfractions of lipoproteins,
    and in their component apolipoproteins?

References

1. Naito KH: Effects of physical activity on serum
    cholesterol metabolism. Cleve Clin Q 43:21, 1976

2. Wood PD, Haskell WL: The effect of exercise on
    plasma high density lipoproteins. Lipids 14:417,
    1979

3. Holloszy JO, Skinner JS, Toro G, Cureton TK: Ef-
    fects of a six-month program of endurance exercise
    on the serum lipids of middle-aged man. Am J Cardiol
    14:753, 1964

4. Lopez-SA, Vial R, Balart L, Arroyave G: Effect of
    exercise and physical fitness on serum lipids and
    lipoproteins. Atherosclerosis 20:1, 1974

5. Wood PW, Haskell WL, Stern MP, Lewis S, Perry C:
    Plasma lipoprotein distributions in male and female
    runners. Ann NY Acad Sci 301:748, 1977

6. Bjorntorp P, Fahlen M, Grimby G, et al: Carbohydrate
    and lipid metabolism in middle-aged, physically
    well-trained men. Metabolism 21:1037, 1972

7. Martin RP, Haskell WL, Wood PD. Blood chemistry and lipid profiles of elite distance runners. Ann NY Acad Sci 301:346, 1977

8. Hurter R, Swale J, Peyman MA, et al: Some immediate and long-term effects of exercise on plasma lipids. Lancet 2:671, 1972

9. Epstein L, Miller GJ, Stitt FW, Morris JN: Vigorous exercise in leisure time, coronary risk factors and resting electrocardiogram in middle-aged male civil servants. Br Med J 38:403, 1976

10. Enger SC, Herbjornsen K, Erikssen J, Fretland A: High density lipoproteins (HDL) and physical activity: the influence of physical activity, age and smoking on HDL-cholesterol and the HDL-/total cholesterol ratio. Scand J Clin Lab Invest 37:251, 1977

11. Lehtonen A, Viikari J: Serum triglycerides and cholesterol and serum high-density lipoprotein cholesterol in highly physically active men. Acta Med Scand 204:111, 1978

12. Lehtonen A, Viikari J: The effect of vigorous physical activty at work on serum lipids with a special reference to serum high-density lipoprotein cholesterol. Acta Physiol Scand 104:117, 1978

13. Montoye HJ, Block WD, Gayle R: Maximal oxygen uptake and blood lipids. J Chron Dis 31:111, 1978

14. Haskell WL, Heiss H: HDL-cholesterol, treadmill exercise test response and strenuous physical activity: LRC prevalence study (abstr). AHA Epidemiology Newsletter 1:72, 1979

15. Mann GV, Garret HL, Farhi A, et al: Exercise to prevent coronary heart disease. Am J Med 46:21, 1969

16. Altekreuse EB, Wilmore J: Changes in blood chemistries following a controlled exercise program. J Occupational Med 15:110, 1973

17. Campbell DE: Influence of several physical activities on serum cholesterol concentration in young men. J Lipid Res 6:478, 1965

18. Melish J, Bronstein D, Gross R, et al: Effect of exercise training in type II hyperlipoproteinemia (abstr). Circulation 58:38, 1978.

19. Carlson LA, Froberg SO: Blood lipids and glucose
     levels during a ten-day period of low-calorie intake
     and exercise in man. Metabolism 16: 624, 1967

20. Weltman A, Stamford BA, Levy RS, et al: Diet, exer-
     cise and lipoprotein cholesterol (abstr). Circula-
     tion 58:204, 1978

21. Carlson LA, Mossefeldt F: Acute effect of prolonged
     heavy exercise on the concentration of plasma lipids
     and lipoprotein in man. Acta Physiol Scand 62:51,
     1964

22. Milesis C: Effects of metered physical training on
     serum lipids of adult men. J Sports Med 14:13, 1974

23. Ratliff R, Elliott K, Rubenstein C: Plasma lipid
     and lipoprotein changes with chronic changes. Med
     Sci Sports 10:55, 1973

24. Oscai LB, Patterson JA, Bogard DL, et al: Normali-
     zation of serum triglycerides and lipoprotein elec-
     trophoretic patterns of exercise. Am J Cardiol
     30:775, 1972

25. Gyntelberg F, Brennan R, Holloszy JO: Plasma tri-
     glyceride lowering by exercise despite increased
     food intake in patients with type II hyperlipopro-
     teinemia. Am J Clin Nutr 30:716, 1977

26. Lampman RM, Santinga JT, Hodge NF: Effectiveness of
     unsupervised and supervised high intensity physical
     training in normalizing serum lipids in men with
     type IV hyperlipoproteinemia. Circulation 57:172,
     1978

27. Nikkila EA, Taskinen M-R, Rehunen S, Harkonen M:
     Lipoprotein lipase activity in adipose and skeletal
     muscle of runners: relation to serum lipoproteins.
     Metabolism 27:1661, 1978

28. Borensztajn J, Rone MS, Babirak SP, McGarr J, Oscai
     L: Effect of exercise on lipoprotein lipase activity
     in rat heart and skeletal muscle. J Physiol 229:394,
     1975

29. Erkelens DW, Albers JJ, Hazzard WR, Frederick RC,
     Bierman EL: Moderate exercise increases high den-
     sity lipoprotein cholesterol in myocardial infarc-
     tion survivors. Clin Res, Vol 26:158A, 1978

30. Miller GJ, Miller NE: Plasma high density lipopro-
     tein concentration and development of ischemic
     heart disease. Lancet 1:16, 1975

31. Williams P, Robinson D, Bailey A: High density lipo-
    protein and coronary risk factors in normal men.
    Lancet 1:72, 1979

32. Carlson LA: Plasma lipids and atherosclerosis: J
    Clin Pathol 26 (suppl) 5:43, 1973

33. Hartung GH, Foreyt JP, Mitchell RE, et al: Rela-
    tionship of diet and HDL-cholesterol in sedentary
    and active middle-aged men. Circulation 58: 204,
    1978

34. Dale E, Gerlach DH, Martin DE, Alexander CR: Physi-
    cal fitness profiles and reproductive physiology of
    the female distance runner. Phys Sports Med 6:83,
    1979

35. Leon AS, Conrad J, Hunninglake D, Jacobs D, Serfass
    R: Exercise effects on body composition, work capa-
    city and carbohydrate and lipid metabolism of young
    obese men. Med Sci Sports 9:60, 1977

36. Krauss RM, Lindgren FT, Wood PD, Haskell WL, Albers
    JJ, Cheung MC: Differential increases in plasma
    high density lipoprotein subfractions and apolipo-
    proteins in runners (abstr). Circulation 56:111,
    1977

37. Nikkila EA, Tuskinen M-R, Rehunen S, Harkoven M:
    Lipoprotein lipase activity in adipose tissue and
    skeletal muscle of runners: relation to serum lipo-
    proteins. Metabolism 27:1661, 1978

38. Simko V, Kelley RE: Increase in plasma lecithin-
    cholesterol acyltransferase (LCAT) and decrease of
    red blood cell (RBC) lipids by physical exercise in
    rats. Am J Clin Nutr 29:482, 1976

39. Schwartz CC, Halloran LG, Vlahcevic ZR, Gregory DH,
    Swell L: Preferential utilization of free choles-
    terol from high density lipoproteins of biliary
    cholesterol secretion in man. Science 200:62, 1978

40. Halloran LG, Schwartz CC, Vlahcevic ZR, Nisman RM,
    Swell L: Evidence for high density lipoprotein-free
    cholesterol as the primary precursor for bile-acid
    synthesis in man. Surgery 84:1, 1978

SUMMARY: PART 2

Jere H. Mitchell, M.D.

Chapter by Blomqvist and Lewis

Maximal oxygen uptake or aerobic work capacity is a
determination of the maximal movement of oxygen from the
ambient air to the tissues of the body. This includes
the ability of the cardiorespiratory system to deliver
oxygen and the capacity of the tissues, particularly
skeletal muscle, to take up oxygen. There is ample evidence that the lungs are not the limiting factor; therefore, the limit must be imposed by the central circulation or the skeletal muscle. Currently there is some
disagreement concerning the limiting role of these two
factors and the relative role of each in the cardiovascular changes that occur with training. Aerobic work
capacity has a significant genetic component; but age,
sex, and habitual level of physical activity are the
most important factors in normal subjects.

Many studies have been done on the cardiovascular
changes that occur from physical training in normal subjects and in patients with ischemic heart disease. In
both of these groups, it has been clearly demonstrated
that such a training program will increase maximal oxygen
uptake.

In both cross-sectional and longitudinal studies on
the effects of endurance training in normal subjects, it
has been shown that the marked differences in maximal
oxygen uptake are due to differences in maximal stroke
volume and cardiac output. Changes in maximal heart rate
and maximal A-VO$_2$ differences are much less important.

In studies of patients with ischemic heart disease
there is some controversy on the relative roles of an

increased stroke volume and an increased A-VO$_2$ difference
in the higher maximal oxygen uptake obtained by training.
One of the most important changes that occurs with physical training is the response to submaximal exercise
loads. At a given level of oxygen uptake, there is a
smaller increase in heart rate and systolic blood pressure. This results in a decreased oxygen need by the
heart for a given level of total body oxygen uptake.
This is of great importance in patients with ischemic
heart disease.

Discussion of Blomqvist and Lewis

There is some controversy concerning the effects of
endurance training on the dimensions and the function of
the left ventricle. It has been shown in cross-sectional
studies of normal subjects and endurance athletes that
the athletes have larger left ventricular volumes and
masses. However, the results of longitudinal studies of
endurance training have not been consistent. Echocardiographic measurements in some studies have shown no change
and in others an increase in left ventricular volume and
mass. This is also true of studies on the contractile
state, some showing no change and some showing an increase. It should also be noted that in many studies
before and after training the measurements are made at
rest and not during exercise.

The effect of training on the autonomic nervous system
may be of some importance. It would appear that the sympathetic drive is less at rest and during submaximal
workloads. This would be important because the relative
bradycardia and lower contractile state would reduce
myocardial oxygen demands. However, at maximal workloads
it appears that there is no reduction in sympathetic
drive after endurance training.

There is interesting data, however, suggesting that
the response of cardiac muscle to catecholamines is increased by training. This may be due to an increase in
the number of beta-adrenergic receptors. Also the effects of training on the central nervous system and the
resultant traffic in sympathetic efferent fibers may
influence receptor sites in the cardiovascular system.

The effect of endurance training on the cardiovascular
system is a complex phenomenon including multiple adaptive
changes at several levels. More basic studies are needed
to unravel these important and fascinating changes that
occur with endurance training.

Myocardial oxygen demand is principally determined by wall stress, heart rate, and contractile state. During dynamic exercise these are all increased and the coronary circulation must provide an adequate oxygen supply to meet this increased metabolic demand. In normal subjects this is principally accomplished by an increase in coronary blood flow with only a modest increase in $A-VO_2$ difference. A useful hemodynamic index of the myocardial oxygen requirement is the product of peak systolic pressure and heart rate ("double product").

With physical training the double product (myocardial oxygen demand) is lower for any given level of submaximal work (body oxygen consumption). Also it has been shown that a patient with ischemic heart disease can get a higher double product after a training program.

More information is needed concerning myocardial perfusion and performance during exercise and endurance training.

Discussion of Klocke and Ellis

In patients the ST segment depression, which is thought to express an imbalance of myocardial oxygen supply and demand, often is greater during recovery after exercise when the heart rate and blood pressure are markedly decreasing. This may be due to a transmural "steal" in which the endocardium is at a relatively greater risk during recovery. It also should be stated that the cuff blood pressure is a reflection of lateral wall pressure and may not indicate changes in coronary perfusion pressure.

The double product is a useful clinical measure of the myocardial oxygen demand. It has been used extensively in the evaluation of patients with coronary heart disease and in the response to therapy in these patients. The double product is a good measure of total left ventricular myocardial oxygen consumption but may not be useful with regional myocardial ischemia. Regional myocardial ischemia may better be evaluated by abnormalities in wall motion.

Coronary flow occurs predominantly during diastole, but during exercise there is a significant systolic component. It is conceivable that myocardial bridging of a coronary artery with delayed reopening might extend into diastole and therefore cause ischemia. Some of the reported cases appear to have generalized left ventricular hypertrophy which may account for the ischemic changes.

Chapter by Haskell

Epidemiological studies have suggested that a high level of total blood cholesterol is a major risk factor for the development of coronary heart disease. Recently it has been suggested that a low level of high density lipoprotein cholesterol (HDL-C) is also a risk factor. A higher level of physical activity, per se, appears to have little effect on the level of total blood cholesterol. However, if the increased physical activity is accompanied by weight loss then a reduction in total blood cholesterol may occur. Also, the level of low density lipoprotein cholesterol (LDL-C) is little affected. Increased physical activity does appear to reduce both plasma triglycerides and very low density lipoprotein cholesterol (VLDL-C).

HDL-C appears to be increased by a higher level of physical activity. This has been shown in both cross-sectional and longitudinal studies. Some, but not all, of these changes are due to differences in adiposity, smoking habits, and alcohol intake. The lower triglycerides and higher HDL-C with increased physical activity may be due to an increase in lipoprotein lipase activity in skeletal muscle or in adipose tissue. The alteration of blood lipids occurring with increased physical activity may be important in reducing the risk of coronary heart disease.

Discussion of Haskell

It must be pointed out that most studies of the effect of physical activity on HDL-C have not considered differences in alcohol intake, which now have been reported to increase HDL-C. However, in the Stanford study, there was no difference in HDL-C levels in runners who were teetotalers and those who consumed large amounts of alcohol.

It is of interest that the relationship between HDL-C and alcohol consumption is a linear one to very high levels of intake while the relationship between alcohol consumption and incidence of coronary heart diseases appears to be a U-shaped one in which there is a high risk with no alcohol consumption, a low risk with moderate alcohol consumption, and a high risk with a high alcohol consumption.

It has been shown in a recent Scandinavian study that a moderate exercise program carried out for 12 weeks can increase the HDL-C approximately 30 percent. In this study there was appropriate control of diet, smoking, and alcohol intake.

The mechanism by which increased physical activity enhances lipoprotein lipase activity has not been worked out. Also, the mechanism by which an increased lipoprotein lipase activity raises the HDL-C is not understood. More studies need to be done in this area.

The changes that are occurring in the concentration of HDL-C with increased physical activity are small. It seems unlikely that such a small change would have any effect on the occurrence of atherosclerosis; however these changes are of the same magnitude that have been shown in epidemiological studies to have a so-called protective effect. Also, it may be that the ratio of LDL-C to HDL-C is a more important number to look at in terms of susceptibility to atherosclerosis.

There have been no studies to date showing that a change in HDL-C has any effect on subsequent atherosclerotic events. Such prospective studies are needed to answer this important point.

General Discussion

It was pointed out that it has not been proven that the level of HDL-C plays any role in the development of atherosclerosis. Therefore, it is premature to speak of the "protective value" of a high level of HDL-C. It would be important to show that changes in the level of HDL-C affect the LDL-C receptor sites.

In future studies it will be important to determine the unique effect of increased physical activity on all of the plasma lipoproteins and to determine what levels of endurance training are needed to bring about these changes. Also, it will be important to determine the mechanisms responsible for these changes in plasma lipoproteins and to establish whether or not there is an association between specific lipoprotein levels and atherosclerotic events.

A study from NHLBI found a decrease in total blood cholesterol with endurance training in subjects who had a high level, but no changes in those who had a normal or low level. Also, when diet and weight changes were controlled, training caused no changes in HDL-C.

At this time it would appear that increased physical activity may not have the same effect in all individuals. If an experimental subject or patient has a low percentage of body fat, is reasonably active, and has a low total blood cholesterol and triglyceride, then a training program may have little effect. At the other extreme, for an individual with abnormal lipoproteins who has a high percentage of body fat and is sedentary, a training program may have a profound effect. Studies to look at the behavior of HDL-C in these separate types need to be investigated.

It appears that endurance training has important effects on the autonomic nervous sytem in both normal subjects and patients. Many patients who are placed in rehabilitation programs are taking beta-adrenergic receptor blocking drugs. A recent study has shown that a cardiovascular training effect can be produced in normal subjects who are taking propranolol. A similar study needs to be done in patients with coronary heart disease.

PART 3

7
RESULTS OF PHYSICAL CONDITIONING IN HEALTHY MIDDLE-AGED SUBJECTS

Henry L. Taylor, Ph.D.

The relationship of physical inactivity to future coronary heart disease (CHD) has been examined in more than 50 population-based reports since Morris et al.[1] first reported on the London busmen 26 years ago. The results of all this work have been extensively discussed and reviewed. In 1972, Froelicher and Oberman[2] concluded in an extensive review that population studies do not establish inactivity as a risk factor of a magnitude comparable to hypercholesterolemia, cigarette smoking, and hypertension.

Froelicher and Oberman described the evidence as both contradictory and inconclusive, citing poorly standardized methods of characterizing the level of habitual activity and the medical status to identify cases of coronary heart disease, as well as the frequent absence of measurements of the established risk factors to control these confounding variables.

In the 5 years following the Froelicher and Oberman review, several developments of interest in this field occurred. Morris and his colleagues[3] published their study of British civil servants using a carefully pretested questionnaire which took advantage of the skills and training of British civil servants to provide information on leisure time activities which could be characterized by the intensity of the activity. The results documented the concept that protection against CHD may well require a relatively intense activity. The only established risk factor used to characterize the participants was the habit of smoking cigarettes. It was shown that the observed relationship of physical activity to future CHD was not dependent on smoking.

In addition, Paffenbarger and his colleagues published several papers on his on-going study of the San Francisco longshoremen.[3,5] The tendency of men in jobs requiring heavy activity to change to more sedentary occupations and the increasing use of labor-saving devices--resulting in major reductions in energy expenditure--were taken into account by Paffenbarger in the analysis of the effects of vigorous work on future CHD. It is well known that men with disease tend to transfer to jobs requiring less energy expenditure, or go into disability retirement. This problem was recognized by Paffenbarger, who did not charge any event which occurred in the first six months after transfer to the lower activity level. It is not clear that this period was long enough to prevent an artificial concentration of CHD events in the low activity group.

There were other develpments which bolstered the concept that exercise is useful in promoting health and is inversely related to coronary heart disease.

For example, the observation by Wood and his colleagues[6] that HDL cholesterol was increased by vigorous exercise took on considerable importance when it was reported by a large collaborative study that HDL cholesterol was inversely related to future CHD.[7] A second biochemical effect of exercise which could be construed to be beneficial and potentially related to future CHD was the demonstration that exercise increased cellular sensitivity to insulin, particularly in the obese, and thus reduced requirements at any given glucose load.[8] Dr. Jean Mayer and his colleagues[9,10] have reported studies in animals and man relating exercise to the control of obesity. Tyroler and the Evans County group of investigators[11] have shown that weight change over time in a freeliving population is related to the blood pressure level. Finally, Paffenbarger has reported that physically active college students had lower blood pressures in middle age.[12]

These developments led Leon and Blackburn[13] to take a somewhat different position in their review of this subject in 1977. The beneficial adaptations to exercise were emphasized, and exercise was recommended as a prudent addition to a hygienic program of CHD prevention in middle-aged men emphasizing reduction of dietary saturated fat, elimination of smoking, and treatment of elevated blood pressure.

The analysis of the 10-year followup of the Seven Countries Study [14] has been completed, and the results should be considered here.

The men were placed in one of three categories of physical activity at entry by occupational titles and a few simple questions. These categories were discussed with local physicians before the initial survey was begun.

Table 1 presents the death rates from coronary heart disease in seven areas where men classed as sedentary could be compared with men engaged in hard work. (Table 3 presents denominators for tables 1 and 2.) In all of the seven areas, the death rate from coronary heart disease was smaller in those engaged in heavy activity than in those engaged in sedentary activity. But in only three of the group was the difference significant. In all of the cohorts listed in table 1, the incidence of "hard CHD" (CHD death plus myocardial infarction) was determined. In six of the cohorts, the incidence of CHD in 10 years for the heavy activity group was numerically less than that of the sedentary group. But only in rural Italy, Rome Railroad, and Zutphen were observed differences statistically significant.

The U.S. Railroad Study was not included in table 1 since the design focused on men in sedentary occupations (executives, dispatchers, and clerks) and one moderately active occupation (switchmen). Switchmen are in the moderately active category in the Seven Countries activity classification. The comparison of death rates in groups with sedentary and moderate activity is presented in table 2. Yugoslavia has a significant difference in the expected direction. But this is a very mixed signal since in Finland the rate of CHD deaths rose from 399 in the sedentary group to 985 in the moderately active group. This difference had a p value of 0.08 which is beginning to approach significance and should be evaluated in light of the fact that the incidence for hard coronary heart disease rose from 708 per 100,000 to 1,621, resulting in a difference whose p value was 0.05. In Yugoslavia there were no CHD deaths in 313 men classed as moderately active, a fact which resulted in a significant difference in the CHD death rates of the sedentary and moderately active group. The hard CHD rates were consistent with this finding. In rural Italy, the CHD death rate of the moderately active men was not different from that of the sedentary men, but the rate for hard CHD did reach significance.

The difference between hard CHD incidence rates of sedentary men and those who were classed as doing hard work reached significance only in the Japanese cohort.

Finally, Keys examined physical activity along with other risk factors as a predictor of future heart disease using the Walker Duncan method of computing probability of developing coronary heart disease by the multiple logistic. For this purpose, the sedentary group was coded 1, the moderately active group, 2, and the group performing hard work, 3. The risk factors which were

Table 1: The Seven Countries Study

Ten Year Age-Adjusted Coronary Heart Disease Deaths in Men Aged 40 to 59 and Cardiovascular Disease-Free at Entry

Cohort	Physical Activity Class			
	Sedentary	Heavy Activity		p
Finland	399	367	-32	-
Rural Italy	500	140	-360	0.001
Rome Railroad	506	131	-375	0.02
Zutphen	359	47	-302	0.06
Yugoslavia	232	153	-79	0.16
Greece	167	16	-151	0.06
Japan	77*	54	-23	-

Data rearranged from Keys[14].

*Sedentary and moderate activity combined.

"-" indicates p>0.25.

N=10,000.

Table 2: The Seven Countries Study

Ten Year Age-Adjusted Coronary Heart Disease Deaths in Men Aged 40 to 59 and Cardiovascular Disease-Free at Entry

Cohort	Physical Activity Class			
	Sedentary	Moderately Active		p
U.S. railroad	416	470	+54	-
Finland	399	985	+586	0.08
Rome railroad	506	196	-310	0.07
Rural Italy	500	194	-306	0.07
Zutphen	359	326	-33	-
Yugoslavia	232	0	-232	0.004
Greece	167	106	-60	-

Data rearranged from Keys[14].

"-" indicates p>0.25.

N=10,000.

Table 3: The Seven Countries Study

Numbers of Men Aged 40 to 59 and Cardiovascular Disease-Free at Entry

Cohort	Physical Activity Class		
	Sedentary	Moderately Active	Heavy Activity
U.S. Railroad	1305	813	-
Finland	147	226	1161
Rome Railroad	161	290	276
Rural Italy	154	370	1139
Zutphen	197	552	96
Yugoslavia	341	313	1187
Greece	208	106	576
Japan	*	*	649

Data rearranged from Keys[14].

*Sedentary and moderate activity combined.

N = 349.

used in the evaluation of physical activity were age, systolic blood pressure, serum cholesterol, smoking habit, and resting pulse rate. The relationship of physical activity recorded at entry to the incidence of death or major coronary heart disease was evaluated by the t value of the coefficient of physical activity in the multiple logistic. The prior hypothesis that CHD incidence was inversely related to the physical activity level was assumed.

The analysis was carried out on the three groups: 1) the American railroad population, 2) the northern European population, and 3) the southern European population.

In the U.S. Railroad Study, the t value of the physical activity coefficient for CHD deaths was very close to zero. The population designated as northern Europe consisted of Finland and Zutphen (Holland). In this group, physical activity was inversely related to CHD deaths and hard CHD by coefficients whose t values were clearly not significant. Finally, in the third group designated as southern Europe, the t value of the coefficient relating physical activity to CHD death was -2.5 (p = 0.01). On the other hand, physical activity was inversely related to the hard CHD endpoint, but the coefficient was not significantly greater than zero. A further report on the U.S. Railroad data, including leisure physical activity, is in preparation.

The univariate within-country or occupation analysis gives a picture of inconsistent results. Inspection of table 3, which presents the numbers by cohort and activity level, reveals low numbers of men classified as sedentary. This raises the possibility of false negative results in some cohorts. Pooling the data by region and applying the multiple logistic appears to have solved the number problem for one endpoint (CHD death) in southern Europe but not in northern Europe. Blackburn[16] has suggested that the protective effect of habitual physical activity may not be great in the presence of overwhelming levels of other risk characteristics in the population.

It can be argued that the effect of exercise on the Finns, who have the highest cholesterol counts in the world, could be overwhelmed by extensive, advanced atherosclerosis. The positive effect found in the southern Europeans--in studies controlled for the effects of cholesterol concentration, blood pressure, smoking habit, resting pulse rate, and age--is impressive because the relationship is independent of the other major risk factors. The difference in the results between northern and southern Europe could be explained by Blackburn's suggestion. But why, then, does the relationship with physical activity fail to reach significance when the hard CHD end point is employed in the southern European group? Invoking the concept that physical activity protected against sudden death in the south but not in the north to explain the discrepancy without supporting evidence is carrying the argument too far. Thus, this difference remains unexplained.

The U.S. Railroad Study was confined to two levels of physical activity required by the occupation. There were men employed as executives, dispatchers, and clerks who were classed as sedentary. In addition, there were switchmen who were classed as moderately active, working in the classification yards and the delivery of freight cars to industry. The occupational energy expenditure of these two groups has been investigated and will be reported in detail elsewhere. Here we summarize the results. The oxygen cost of each task required of these men was measured in the field. Time spent at each task over an 8-hour shift was measured and calories expended during the work shift were calculated. On the average during an 8-hour shift, switchmen expended 375 calories more than the clerks did. In addition, a dietary survey was conducted on a small sample (N = 33). Food was weighed in the home. For a 24-hour day, switchmen consumed 510 calories more than the clerks.

All men who were not disqualified on medical grounds were submitted to a submaximal 3-minute exercise test. Mean work pulse rates of switchmen were 10 beats a minute less than the mean of the clerks and other sedentary individuals. Oxygen pulse was determined in a Minneapolis subsample, and the difference between switchmen and clerks persisted. The numbers of men studied were adequate so there seems little likelihood that this is a false negative result. It is concluded that the cardiovascular conditioning of the switchmen was higher than that of the clerks.

The conclusion reached by Keys is that the Seven Countries data on physical activity as a risk factor are inconsistent. This is clearly the conservative scientific position. It is concluded here that simply improving the cardiovascular conditioning of a sedentary man is not enough to provide him with significant protection against CHD. These data support the concept advanced by Blackburn[16] that a threshold of physical activity is required which is greater than roughly 300 calories a day if, indeed, physical activity does protect against coronary disease.

A major problem in the interpretation of prospective studies of risk factors for coronary heart disease which include physical activity as a variable to be evaluated is that of selection. Suppose that at the end of such a study, physical activity was shown to be associated with the development of future coronary heart disease and

116

that this association is still significant while control-
ling for the established risk factors. One is then left
with the problem of whether the physical activity itself
provided the beneficial result, or whether those who
elected to take jobs requiring heavy activity or elected
to take up a sport such as cross-country skiing brought
along with them personal characteristics which protected
them from the lethal effects of atherosclerosis. There
appears to be no way to solve this problem other than to
run a controlled trial with subjects randomly assigned
to control and treatment groups.

A randomized trial has the advantage of eliminating
questions regarding selection and providing hard data on
the amount of exercise engaged in by the subjects. Furthermore, medical examinations at regular intervals and
regular contact with the staff and with the participant's
physician provide the data for precise classification of
end points. In short, the randomized trial provides the
opportunity to settle many of the uncertainties which now
hang over the evaluation of physical inactivity as a risk
factor.

Some years ago, we were associated with a study of the
feasibility of mounting such a controlled trial in middle-
aged men. Middle-aged males were randomly assigned to
control and experimental groups for an 18-month study.[17]
We found that the rate of adherence to the exercise
prescription dropped off after 6 months to 50 percent.
A similar result was obtained by a comparable study in
Finland.[18] This translates into a very large sample
size and heavy expense for facilities, equipment, and
supervisory personnel. The conclusion was that such a
trial in high risk, but otherwise healthy middle-aged
men, was not feasible.

On the other hand, the sample size for a trial of physical activity in the rehabilitation of post-myocardial
infarction patients is not out of reach because of the
high reinfarction rate. It is believed that such a trial
would make a contribution to our understanding of the
role of exercise in the prevention of coronary heart
disease.

An examination of those adaptations to exercise which
are potentially related to both the prolongation of life
in the post-myocardial infarction patient and the development of future CHD in normals is presented in table 4.
These effects and the variables concerned are well known.
Of the six adaptations listed, five can be monitored.
Of these five, two will be monitored in a minimal design.
The addition of measures of blood coagulation and fibrinolysis, plasma insulin concentration, and plasma HDL and
triglyceride would not appear to be unnecessarily burden-
some. It is reasonable to assume that a majority of the

Table 4: Postulated Mechanisms in CHD Prevention by Exercise

---

1. A reduction in work heart rate and blood pressure (at given level of work) resulting in a reduction of myocardial oxygen requirements for any given amount of work.

2. Possible increased myocardial vascularity including capillary density, coronary collaterals, and size of coronary artery tree.

3. Reduced blood coagulability and a transient increase in fibrinolysis.

4. Reduction in weight and adiposity.

5. Increased cellular sensitivity to insulin reducing insulin requirements at any given glucose load.

6. A reduction in triglycerides and an increase in HDL in the blood.

---

post-myocardial infarction patients in a supervised exercise program will work hard enough to modify a majority of these variables. The Coronary Drug Project learned a great deal regarding prediction of survival of post-myocardial infarction patients.[19,20] Since these predictors come principally from the electrocardiogram and the medical history, the data to control for prognostic differences between individuals should be available again without undue expense. The effects of modifications of the exercise variables can then be related to survival.

A carefully designed controlled trial in post-myocardial infarction patients will make a contribution to our understanding of exercise and coronary heart disease. If successful, it will reinforce the relatively soft data we have on exercise and the development of CHD in normals. Monitoring indicators of potential mechanisms for benefit may produce important etiologic evidence within the control and treatment groups. A trial of rehabilitation of post-myocardial infarction patients is suggested for these reasons as well as to help answer the primary question: Does exercise prolong survival?

References

1. Morris JN, Heady JA, Raffle PAB, Roberts CG, Parks JW: Coronary heart disease and physcial activity of work. Lancet 256:1053-1057, 1111-1120, 1953

2. Froelicher VD, Oberman A: Analysis of epidemiologic studies of physical inactivity as risk factor for coronary artery disease. Prog Cardiovasc Dis 15: 41-65, 1972

3. Morris JN, Chave SPW, Adam C, Sirey C, Epstein L, Sheehan DJ: Vigorous exercise in leisure time and the incidence of coronary heart disease. Lancet i:333-339, 1973

4. Paffenbarger RS Jr, Gima AS, Laughlin ME, Mary E, Black RA: Characteristics of longshoremen related to CHD and stroke. Am J Public Health 61:13621370, 1971

5. Paffenbarger RS Jr, Hale WE: Work activity and coronary heart mortality. N Engl J Med 292:545-550, 1975

6. Wood PD, Klein PD, Lewis S, Haskell WL: Plasma lipoprotein concentrations in middle-aged male runners (abstr). Circulation 49 (suppl 3):115, 1974

7. Castelli WP, Doyle JT, Gordon T, Haines CG, Mjortland MC, Hulley SB, Kagan A, Zukel WJ: HDL cholesterol and other lipids in coronary heart disease--the cooperative lipoprotein phenotyping study. Circulation 55:767, 1977

8. Bjorntorp BP, Fahlen M, Grimby G, Gustafson A, Holm J, Renstrom P, Schersten T: Carbohydrate and lipid metabolism and middle-aged physically well trained men. Metabolism 21:1037-1044, 1972

9. Mayer J: Exercise, food intake, and body weight in normal rats and genetically obese adult mice. Am J Physiol 177:544, 1954

10. Mayer J, Ray P, Mitra RP: Relation between caloric intake, body weight, and physical work. Studies in an industrial male population in West Bengal. Am J Clin Nutr 4:169, 1956

11. Tyroler HA, Heyden S, Hames CG: Weight and hypertension: Evans County studies of blacks and whites. In, Epidemiology and Control of Hypertension (Paul O, ed). New York, Stratton, 1975, p 177

12. Paffenbarger RS, Thome MC, Wing AL: Chronic disease in former college students. VIII. Characteristics in youth predisposing to hypertension in later years. Am J Epidemiol 88:25, 1968

13. Leon AS, Blackburn H: The relationship of physical activity to coronary heart disease and life expectancy. Ann NY Acad Sci 301:561-579, 1977

14. Keys A: Seven countries--coronary heart disease and deaths in ten years. Cambridge, Harvard Press, January, 1980

15. Taylor HL, Jacobs D, Blackburn H, Keys A: Leisure time and occupational physical activity in selected sedentary and physically active railroad employees (in preparation)

16. Blackburn H: Physical activity and cardiovascular health: the epidemiological evidence. In, Physical Activity and Human Well-being, (Landry, Orban eds). Miami, Symposia Specialists, 1978, p 138

17. Taylor HL, Buskirk ER, Remington RD: Exercise in controlled trials of the prevention of coronary heart disease. Fed Proc 32:1623-1627, 1973

18. Pyorala K, Karava R, Punsar S, Oja P, Teraslinna P, Partanen T, Jaaskelainen M, Pekkarinen M, Koskela A: A controlled study of the effects of 18 months physical training in sedentary middle-aged men with high indices of risk relative to coronary heart disease. In, Coronary Heart Disease and Physical Fitness (Larsen OA, Malmborg RO, eds). Baltimore, University Park Press, 1971, p 265

19. The Coronary Drug Project Research Group: The prognostic importance of the electrocardiogram after myocardial infarction. Experience in the coronary drug project. Ann Intern Med 77:677, 1972

20. The Coronary Drug Project: Factors influencing long-term prognosis after recovery from myocardial infarction--three-year findings of the coronary drug project. J Chron Dis 27:267, 1974

8
THERAPEUTIC EFFECTS OF EXERCISE TRAINING IN ANGINA PATIENTS

Rudolph H. Dressendorfer, Ph.D.
Ezra A. Amsterdam, M.D.
Dean T. Mason, M.D.

Exercise training of the aerobic type results in a number of important physiological alterations of demonstrable or potential benefit to the patient with coronary heart disease, including enhancement of exertional capacity and elevation of the symptom-limited activity threshold.[1] The latter effects have provided a basis for the application of exercise as a form of medical therapy in angina pectoris. Consideration of the pathophysiology of angina affords an understanding of the therapeutic role of exercise in alleviating this syndrome.

Pathophysiology of Angina

Angina is a manifestation of myocardial ischemia that results from a disparity between cardiac oxygen supply and demand due to obstructive coronary artery disease. Treatment of angina is based on alleviation of the metabolic imbalance by increasing myocardial oxygen supply or reducing demand.[2] Recent studies indicate that surgical revascularization of the myocardium increases oxygen delivery and that medical forms of therapy are effective in treating angina by reducing cardiac oxygen requirements.[3]

Supported in part by Program Project Research Grant HL-14780 from the National Heart, Lung, and Blood Institute, National Institutes of Health, Bethesda, Maryland and Research Grants from California chapters of the American Heart Association, Dallas, Texas.

Myocardial oxygen requirements are principally determined by three factors: heart rate, contractility, and wall tension (related to ventricular volume and pressure).[4] Reduction of any of these factors in an optimal manner to decrease myocardial oxygen consumption without impairing cardiac performance allows a greater intensity and duration of exertion before angina occurs. It has been shown that myocardial oxygen consumption, although dependent on these three factors, is closely related to the two most easily obtainable of these variables, heart rate and blood pressure, in terms of their product.[3]

The double product of heart rate times systolic blood pressure thus correlates closely with relative myocardial oxygen consumption during exertion, and the double product at which angina occurs represents an externally measurable threshold for myocardial ischemia that is constant for the individual patient. A reduced exertional heart rate-blood pressure response, which reflects a decrease in myocardial oxygen consumption toward a level compatible with the restricted flow capacity of the impaired coronary circulation, results in a more favorable balance between myocardial oxygen supply and demand; it allows a greater intensity and duration of work prior to attainment of the ischemic threshold. Onset of angina usually does occur, however, when the ischemic threshold is reached.

Therapeutic Actions of Exercise Training

The ability of exercise to alleviate angina and enhance exertional capacity is apparent from study of the pathophysiology of angina and the physiological effects of exercise. Exercise training of the aerobic type produces an increase in physical working capacity and in total peak somatic oxygen consumption and is associated with diminished hemodynamic stress at any given submaximal workload (figure 1).[1] The trained state is characterized by a lowering of heart rate and blood pressure (chiefly the former) at any subanginal physical stress compared to the rate and pressure response in the untrained state.

Requirements for Exercise Training Effects

Achievement of the physiological alterations associated with improvement in cardiovascular functional capacity requires adherence to specific criteria of an

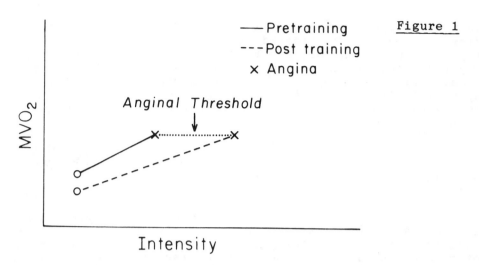

Figure 1

exercise program. The activity must be of the continuous, rhythmic aerobic type. Further, a minimum
threshold of intensity, duration, and frequency of exercise is necessary for improvement of functional capacity.
The exercise prescription is, therefore, based on four
essential factors: type, intensity, duration, and
frequency.[5]

Aerobic activity includes those forms of exercise
involving rhythmic contractions of large muscle groups
continuously working to move the body for prolonged
periods. Examples are walking, jogging, cycling, swimming, skipping rope, rowing, and aerobic dancing. The
minimum intensity of exercise training needed to improve
aerobic capacity is 50 to 60 percent of maximum oxygen
consumption. In coronary patients, lower levels of
intensity may be indicated initially by signs and symptoms
seen after relatively little work. The minimum duration of each exercise session is 10 minutes, but 20 to
30 minutes is preferred. A frequency of three or four
sessions per week is sufficient to achieve a training
effect, provided that intensity and duration of exercise
are adequate.

Screening of the Angina Patient for Exercise Training

Proper selection of patients is the initial step in an
exercise training program. Careful, systematic screening of potential candidates will increase the rate of
successful results, enhance the safety of the program,
and reduce harmful events associated with exercise.
Initial screening eliminates patients at high risk of
such events and assesses motivation in those who qualify

on a medical basis.[6] Conditions judged to be contraindications must be considered in terms of their severity, degree of control, and risk to the patient, requiring individual assessment of circumstances in each
case. Prior to entry in a prescribed exercise program,
symptom-limited exercise testing is mandatory in order
to evaluate the patient's ischemic threshold and aerobic
work tolerance.

Assessment of Functional Aerobic Capacity

Graded exercise testing serves two primary objectives
in the evaluation of the angina patient's functional
capacity. First, the test gradually increases myocardial
oxygen demand ($M\dot{V}O_2$) to the point of ischemic electrocardiographic change and onset of angina pectoris--the
angina threshold (the point of myocardial oxygen supply-
demand imbalance) as determined indirectly by multiplying
the heart rate by the systolic blood pressure (rate-pressure product).[3]

Second, the peak external workload or total somatic
oxygen consumption ($\dot{V}O_2$) achieved may be used to quantify
the patient's aerobic work tolerance (table 1). Thus,

Table 1: Typical Range of Oxygen Consumption ($\dot{V}O_2$)
Values at Peak Treadmill Exercise in Middle-aged,
Sedentary Men and Coronary Patients Before Aerobic
Training

	Oxygen Consumption ml/kg/min	METs	Reason for Test Termination
Untrained normals	28-35	8-10	General fatigue
Coronary patients			
Healed myocardial infarction*	21-28	6-8	Leg fatigue
Post-bypass surgery*	21-28	6-8	Leg fatigue
Angina	7-21	2-6	Angina pectoris

*Uncomplicated, no angina.

the graded cycle ergometer or treadmill test places progressively greater demands on the oxygen supply mechanisms

of both the myocardium and the active skeletal muscles, until the functional limitation is reached. In the angina patient in particular, myocardial oxygen supply becomes insufficient well before peripheral oxygen deprivation limits further exercise. Consequently, when assessing the functional status of the angina patient, it is essential to distinguish between the work capacity of the exercising muscles and symptom limitations caused by inability to satisfy $M\dot{V}O_2$, i.e., the work level at the point of exercise-limiting angina is usually well below the patient's potential maximum performance. In contrast, the normal individual is able to increase $\dot{V}O_2$ to a plateau level of maximum oxygen consumption ($\dot{V}O_2$ max), at which point further exercise is limited by skeletal muscle fatigue due to inadequate arterial oxygen delivery (figure 2).

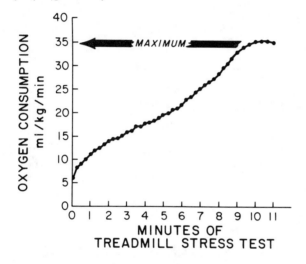

Figure 2

Figure 3 shows the relationship we have observed between the subjective rating of perceived exertion[7] and directly-measured $\dot{V}O_2$ in graded treadmill exercise tests of normal untrained men and of men with angina pectoris.[8] Whereas in healthy individuals the test is terminated upon volitional fatigue at ratings above "hard," the angina patient is typically limited by chest pain to significantly lower levels of perceived exertion. This difference in perceived muscular effort at maximum work tolerance indicates that limitation of exercise capacity occurs in most angina patients considerably below their potential maximum $\dot{V}O_2$.

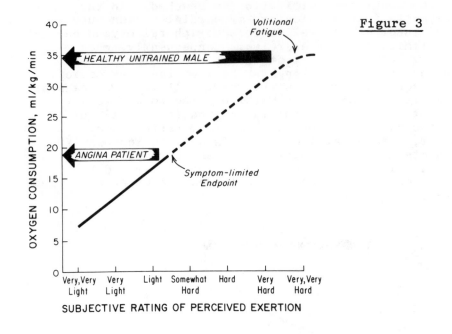

Figure 3

The peak $\dot{V}O_2$ of age-matched angina patients averages only about 50 percent of the normal percentage of $\dot{V}O_2$ max achieved by healthy men during graded exercise testing plotted against perceived exertion (figure 4).

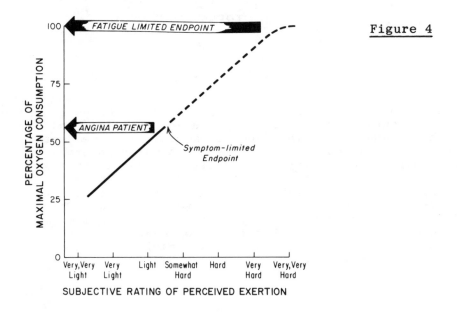

Figure 4

Since arterial lactate concentration remains near resting
levels at exercise intensities below 60 percent of VO_2
max,[9] aerobic energy production is probably not fully
used by the angina patient. Consequently, those observed
physiological adaptations to exercise training that improve functional capacity in subjects with effort-limiting
angina must necessarily be due mainly to aerobic mechanisms related to the oxygen requirements of the heart
and exercising muscles.

Effects of Exercise Training in the Angina Patient

Numerous studies have demonstrated improved functional
aerobic capacity in both pre- and postmyocardial infarction patients with stable angina pectoris following exercise training programs.[10-35] As a result of training,
the majority of patients studied were able to perform
higher external workloads before onset of exercise-limiting anginal pain. Table 2 is a summary of physiological
effects that may elicit improved aerobic work tolerance
in the angina patient.

Table 2: Summary of Known and Postulated Cardiac and
Peripheral Vascular Effects of Exercise Training in
Angina Patients with Improved Aerobic Work Tolerance

	At rest	At fixed workload below angina threshold
Cardiac Effects:		
Heart rate	Decreased	Decreased
Stroke volume	Unchanged or increased*	Unchanged or increased*
Cardiac output	Decreased or unchanged	Decreased
LV systolic pressure	Decreased	Decreased
Contractility	Decreased*	Decreased*
Coronary blood flow	Unchanged	Increased*
Myocardial oxygen demand	Decreased	Decreased
Peripheral Vascular Effects: Effects:		
Blood volume	Increased	Increased
Arterial systolic pressure	Unchanged or decreased	Unchanged or decreased
Arterial oxygen content	Unchanged or increased	Unchanged or increased
Blood flow to exercising muscle		Decreased
Arteriovenous oxygen difference	Increased or unchanged	Increased
Catecholamine levels	Decreased	Decreased
Total somatic oxygen consumption	Unchanged	Decreased

*Postulated.

127

Cardiac and systemic mechanisms postulated to explain increased aerobic work tolerance in subjects with exertional angina are listed in table 3.

Table 3:   Potential Exercise Training Adaptations in Angina Patients to Explain Their Improved Aerobic Work Tolerance

---

Cardiac Mechanisms:

   Improved oxygen supply to ischemic myocardium*

   Improved left ventricular function*

   Raised threshold for perception of anginal pain*

   Decreased myocardial oxygen demand at workloads
      below ischemic threshold***

Systemic Mechanisms:

   Increased oxygen delivery to exercising muscle*

   Greater oxidative capacity of trained muscle**

   Enhanced mechanical efficiency**

Available evidence: *weak or conflicting; **moderate;   ***strong.

Cardiac mechanisms

Improved oxygen supply to ischemic regions of myocardium

In general, there is little evidence to show that coronary blood flow or regional myocardial perfusion is increased by training.[13,14,18,20,27,28] The question of whether training infleunces coronary collateral development nevertheless remains unsolved because of the inability of angiographic techniques to visualize and evaluate collaterals during exercise as well as at rest.   One report has demonstrated, however, that coronary collateral vessel development following experimental coronary occlusion in trained dogs did not enhance regional perfusion of the ischemic myocardium during tachycardia-induced atrial pacing.[20]

Improved left ventricular function

Several angiographic investigations of left ventricular end-diastolic volume and pressure, ejection fraction, and stroke volume have failed to show significant changes following regular exercise training.[19,22,23,25] It is possible that improvement was made but was not detected because the measurements were made with the subjects at rest in the supine position. But in one study,[25] stroke volume during upright exercise at the same percentage of $\dot{V}O_2$ max, measured before and after training, was unchanged. Recent radionuclide angiographic studies made during exercise also failed to detect any significant effect of training on left ventricular function.[36]

Raised threshold for perception of exertional angina

Exercise training has been followed by total relief of reported angina in some patients.[10,17,21,22,24,37] Clearly, functional aerobic capacity will increase when and if the patient becomes less sensitive to anginal pain; in some cases, a corresponding increase did occur in the estimated MVO_2 associated with onset of angina. Following an exercise program, therefore, increased myocardial ischemia may be required in order to produce equivalent perceived anginal pain.[38]

Systemic Mechanisms

Decreased myocardial oxygen demand at workloads below the ischemic threshold

The preponderance of data indicate that physical training improves aerobic work tolerance before the ischemic threshold is attained by reducing $M\dot{V}O_2$ at the same $\dot{V}O_2$.[10-14,16-19,21-31] A higher external workload, then, is required after training in order to produce the same $M\dot{V}O_2$ level that resulted in symptom limitations before training. It should be noted that the reduction in $M\dot{V}O_2$ has not been measured directly but rather hypothesized, based on a significantly lower rate-pressure product, triple product, or tension-time index at given workloads after training. An increase of 10 to 15 percent in the $\dot{V}O_2/HR$ ratio, or oxygen pulse, during exercise—as opposed to decreased rise in systolic blood pressure during exercise—appears to be responsible for most of the lowered $M\dot{V}O_2$ and greater work tolerance.

The antianginal mechanisms of exercise training appear similar in effect to medical therapy, which produces a more favorable balance between myocardial oxygen demand and supply by reducing the former through its actions on heart rate and blood pressure.[2,3] The antianginal actions of the nitrates are a result of their reduction of ventricular volume and systolic blood pressure. The therapeutic actions of beta adrenergic blockade in angina are diminution of heart rate, myocardial contractility, and systolic blood pressure. It should be emphasized that rational antianginal therapy may simultaneously involve more than one form of medical treatment. This combined approach is reflected by the data in table 4,

Table 4: Effect of Therapy on Time to Angina During Graded Exercise Testing in Five Patients

	Control	NTG	Prop	ET	NTG + ET	Prop + NTG + ET
Time to Angina (min)	6.7	9.6*	8.3*	8.5†	10.7†	12.2†

*p <0.05 †p <.005

NTG = nitroglycerin; Prop = propranolol; ET = exercise training.

which demonstrate improved exercise tolerance after medical therapy in five patients with angina after eight weeks of exercise training. Note that combined therapy yielded greater benefit than the individual modes of treatment.

Increased oxygen delivery to exercising muscle

There is no evidence to indicate greater arterial oxygen transport capacity in angina patients following an exercise program. Although blood hemoglobin concentration may increase with training to enhance arterial oxygen content, cardiac output at a given $\dot{V}O_2$ usually decreases in patients with coronary artery disease, due to a lower exercise heart rate.[10,12,13,25] In the angina patient, blood flow to muscles exercising at the same workload probably decreases with training, as suggested by higher arteriovenous oxygen difference,[10,25] reflecting greater peripheral oxygen extraction.

130

Greater oxidative capacity of trained muscle

Skeletal muscle adapts to endurance training by increasing its enzymatic potential for aerobic metabolism.[39] This increased aerobic capacity at the cellular level permits a lower blood flow in trained muscles at a given $\dot{V}O_2$.[10]

Enhanced mechanical efficiency

The ratio of external work output to $\dot{V}O_2$ provides an index of aerobic work efficiency. When this ratio increases, efficiency increases, and greater levels of exercise may be met with unchanged or even reduced total somatic oxygen requirements. It has been shown that, in fact, patients with coronary artery disease improve their exercise tolerance after moderate endurance training by becoming more efficient performers rather than by increasing their aerobic capacity.[40] Further investigation of coronary patients is required in order to document the importance of skill acquisition to total somatic oxygen consumption in physical training.

Major mechanisms of improvement

It is our view that, of the potential mechanisms by which angina patients improve aerobic work tolerance, the available evidence favors reduction of myocardial oxygen demand at subanginal workloads via skeletal muscle adaptation.[10] Enhanced mechanical efficiency also appears to play a contributory role.

Concepts of Adaptation to Exercise Training

The effect of adaptation to exercise training in angina pectoris is a reduction in myocardial oxygen consumption, as measured noninvasively, at a given level of total $\dot{V}O_2$. Figure 5 shows a hypothetical scheme for dual control of $M\dot{V}O_2$ during exercise. The determinants of $M\dot{V}O_2$, i.e., heart rate, wall tension, and myocardial contractility, entail the cardiac response to autonomic innervation via outflow from the vasomotor center, which receives neural input from the exercising muscles ("peripheral drive") and from the motor cortex ("central drive"). Alteration in either the central or peripheral drive will change the balance between sympathetic stimulation and vagal inhibition, and will consequently affect $M\dot{V}O_2$.

It has been shown that aerobic training reduces the peripheral drive during submaximal exercise. This reduction is restricted to exercise using the trained limbs, reflecting the principle of muscle group specificity in

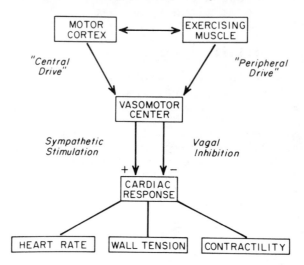

Dual Control of
Myocardial Oxygen Demand During Exercise

Figure 5.

relation to physical training.[10,41,42] Reduced central
drive from the cerebral cortex after training would be
indicated by a lowered $M\dot{V}O_2$ at rest. This conclusion
is predicated upon the existence of insignificant peripheral input to the vasomotor center in the resting
state. Reduced $M\dot{V}O_2$ at rest in the trained patient
must therefore be centrally mediated.

Based on our dual control hypothesis, the relation-
ship between $M\dot{V}O_2$ and $\dot{V}O_2$ is portrayed graphically in
Figure 6. Decreased resting $M\dot{V}O_2$ and a parallel downward shift in the linear increase in $M\dot{V}O_2$ with exercise
would imply reduced central drive. Improved aerobic
work tolerance at the angina threshold, indicated by increased peak $\dot{V}O_2$, results from this downward shift in
$M\dot{V}O_2$ (Figure 6a). If peripheral drive alone were reduced
after training, there would be no change in resting MVO_2
(figure 6b). However, exercise $M\dot{V}O_2$ would be reduced
in a nonparallel fashion because of decreased excitatory
input from the trained muscles during work at a given
total $\dot{V}O_2$.

Combined reduction of central and peripheral drives
would result in a decreased resting $M\dot{V}O_2$ as well as
decreased $M\dot{V}O_2$ during exercise, as shown in figure 6c.
It should be noted that these concepts do not require
alteration in myocardial oxygen supply-demand balance
after training for improvement of aerobic work tolerance

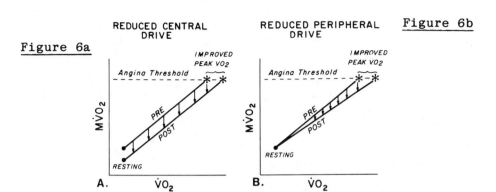

Figure 6a   Figure 6b

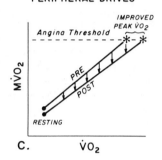

Figure 6c

and are consistent with previous findings of reduced MVO_2 at subanginal effort (figure 1).

Summary

    Exercise training of the aerobic type has augmented exertional capacity and increased the symptom-limited activity threshold in a majority of properly selected angina patients to whom this approach was applied. The antianginal effects of exercise training are similar to those of pharmacologic therapy in that the trained state is characterized by a reduction in myocardial oxygen requirements at subanginal external workloads, thereby improving the myocardial oxygen supply-demand relationship and alleviating ischemia. The reduction of myocardial oxygen demand associated with exercise training is the result of attenuation of the heart rate and, to a lesser degree, the systolic blood pressure response to exertional stress. Achievement of these physiological alterations is dependent on fulfillment of certain minimum criteria by the exercise program, including type of exercise (aerobic), intensity (50 to 60 percent of maximum $\dot{V}O_2$), duration of each session (20 to 30 minutes), and frequency (3 to 4 times per week).

Before initiation of an exercise program, graded exercise testing is necessary in order to determine myocardial ischemic threshold and aerobic work tolerance. A number of structural and functional alterations associated with exercise training appear to contribute to the improved physical capacity in angina patients. The two major mechanisms by which exercise improves aerobic work tolerance in angina appear to be a greater capacity for oxidative metabolism of trained skeletal muscles and enhanced mechanical efficiency of the trained patient for performing physical tasks such as walking.

These factors decrease myocardial oxygen demand at a given total somatic oxygen consumption in the trained compared to the untrained state. A dual control mechanism, consisting of peripheral and central drives, is hypothesized for regulation of myocardial oxygen consumption. Current data support the theory of reduced peripheral and central drives as causing the physiologic and therapeutic effects of exercise training in angina patients.

References

1. Amsterdam EA, Dressendorfer R, Mason DT, Laslett LJ: Exercise training in coronary heart disease: physiological rationale, clinical indications, and practical application. In, Advances in Heart Disease Vol 2 (Mason DT, ed). New York, Grune & Stratton, 1978, pp 345-362

2. Amsterdam EA, Mason DT: Current medical management of angina pectoris. In, Advances in Management of Clinical Heart Disease Vol 2 (Haft, Bailey, eds). Mt Kisco, New York, Futura 1978, pp 237-263

3. Amsterdam EA, Price JE, Berman DS, Hughes JL III, Riggs K, DeMaria AN, Miller RR, Mason DT: Exercise Testing in the indirect assessment of myocardial oxygen consumption: application for evaluation of mechanisms and therapy of angina pectoris. In, Exercise in Cardiovascular Health and Disease (Amsterdam EA, Wilmore JH, DeMaria AN, eds). New York, Yorke Medical Books, 1977, pp 218-233

4. Sonnenblick EH, Ross J Jr, Braunwald E: Oxygen consumption of the heart. Newer concepts of its multifactorial determination. Am J Cardiol 22: 328, 1968

5. Wilmore JH: Individualized exercise prescription. In, Exercise in Cardiovascular Health and Disease (Amsterdam EA, Wilmore JH, DeMaria AN, eds). New York, Yorke Medical Books, 1977, pp 267-273

6. McHenry MM: Medical screening of patients with coronary artery disease: criteria for entrance into exercise conditioning programs (Amsterdam EA, Wilmore JH, DeMaria AN, eds). New York, Yorke Medical Books, 1977, pp 313-321

7. Borg G: Psychological and physiological studies of physical work. In, Measurement of Man at Work (Singleton, Fox, Whitfield, eds). London, Taylor and Francis, 1971, p 121

8. Dressendorfer RH, Amsterdam EA: An approach to preventive cardiology in asymptomatic, sedentary adults. Cardiology 354:1980 (in press)

9. Gollnick PD, Hermansen L: Biochemical adaptations to exercise: anaerobic metabolism. In, Exercise and Sport Sciences Reviews, Vol 1 (Wilmore, ed). New York, Academic Press, 1973

10. Clausen JP: Circulatory adjustments to dynamic exercise and effect of physical training in normal subjects and in patients with coronary artery disease. Progr Cardiovasc Dis 18:459, 1976

11. Clausen JP, Larsen OA, Trap-Jensen J: Physical training in the management of coronary artery disease. Circulation 40:143, 1969

12. Clausen JP, Trap-Jensen J: Effects of training on the distribution of cardiac output in patients with coronary artery disease. Circulation 42:611, 1970

13. Varnauskas E, Bergman H, Houk P, Bjorntorp P: Hemodynamic effects of physical training in coronary patients. Lancet 2:8, 1966

14. Ferguson RJ, Cote P, Gauthier P, Bourassa MG: Changes in exercise coronary sinus blood flow with training in patients with angina pectoris. Circulation 58:41, 1978

15. Hellerstein HK: Exercise therapy in coronary disease. Bull NY Acad Med 44:1028, 1968

16. Frick MH, Katila M: Hemodynamic consequences of physical training after myocardial infarction. Circulation 37:192, 1968

17. Redwood DR, Rosing DR, Epstein SE: Circulatory and symptomatic effects of physical training in patients with coronary-artery disease and angina pectoris. N Engl J Med 286:959, 1972

18. Sim DN, Neill WA: Investigation of the physiological basis for increased exercise threshold for angina pectoris after physical conditioning. J Clin Invest 54:763, 1974

19. Lee AP, Ice R, Blessey R, Sanmarco ME: Long-term effects of physical training on coronary patients with impaired ventricular function. Circulation 60:1519, 1979

20. Neill WA, Oxendine JM: Exercise can promote coronary collateral development without improving perfusion of the ischemic myocardium. Circulation 60:1513, 1979

21. Sanne H: Exercise tolerance and physical training on non-selected patients after myocardial infarction. Acta Med Scand (suppl 1):1, 1973

22. Letac B, Cribier A, Desplanches JF: A study of left ventricular function before and after physical training. Circulation 56:375, 1977

23. Kennedy CC, Spiekerman RE, Lindsay MI Jr, Mankin HT, Frye RL, McCallister BD: One-year graduated exercise program for men with angina pectoris: evaluation by physiologic studies and coronary arteriography. Mayo Clin Proc 51:231, 1976

24. Kavanagh T, Shephard RJ: Conditioning of post-coronary patients: comparison of continuous and interval training. Arch Phys Med Rehab 56:72, 1975

25. Detry J-M, Rousseau R, Vandenbroucke M, Kusumi F, Brasseur LA, Bruce RA: Increased arteriovenous oxygen difference after physical training in coronary disease. Circulation 44:109, 1971

26. Caudus D, Fuentes F, Srinivasan R: Cardiac evaluation of a physical rehabilitation program for patients with ischemic heart disease. Arch Phys Med Rehab 56:419, 1975

27. Fernandez de la Vega Roma PA, Ehsani AA, Holloszy JO, Sobel BE, Hagberg J, Heath G: Results of a prolonged program of physical training in patients with ischemic cardiopathology. Arch Inst Cardiol Mex 48:1161, 1978

28. Ferguson RJ, Petitclerc R, Choquette G, Chaniotis L, Gauthier R, Huot C, Allare L, Jankowski L, Campeau L: Effect of physical training on treadmill exercise capacity, collateral circulation and progression of coronary disease. Am J Cardiol 34:764, 1974

29. Selvester R, Camp J, Sanmarco M: Effects of exercise training on progression of documented coronary arteriosclerosis in men. NY Acad Sci 301:495, 1977

30. Bruce RA, Kusumi F, Frederick R: Differences in cardiac function with prolonged physical training for cardiac rehabilitation. Am J Cardiol 40:597, 1977

31. Cooksey JD, Reilly P, Brown S, Bromze H, Cryer PE: Exercise training and plasma catecholamines in patients with ischemic heart disease. Am J Cardiol 42:372, 1978

32. Oldridge NB, Nagle FJ, Balke B, Corliss RJ, Kahn DR: Aortocoronary bypass surgery: Effects of surgery and 32 months of physical conditioning on treadmill performance. Arch Phys Med Rehab 59:268, 1978

33. Banister EW, Licorish KA, Griffiths J, Taunton JE: Plasma catecholamine changes in response to rehabilitation exercise therapy in post-myocardial infarction patients. Med Sci Sports 5:70, 1973

34. Paterson DH, Shephard RJ, Cunningham D, Jones NL, Andrew G: Effects of physical training on cardiovascular function following myocardial infarction. J Appl Physiol 47:482, 1979

35. Froelicher V, Battler A, McKirnan MD: Physical activity and coronary heart disease. Cardiology 65: 153, 1980

36. Battler A, Froelicher V, Slutsky R, McKirnan D, Strong ML, Ashburn W, Ross J: Initial observations of changes in ventricular function after exercise in coronary disease patients (abstract). Circulation 59 and 60 (II):21, 1979

37. Ehsani AA, Heath GW, Hagberg JM, Holloszy JO: Influence of exercise training on ischemic ST segment response in patients with coronary artery disease (abstract). Circulation 59 and 60 (II):22, 1979

38. Detry JM, Bruce RA: Effects of nitroglycerin on "maximal" oxygen intake and exercise electrocardiogram in coronary heart disease. Circulation 43:155, 1971

39. Holloszy JO: Adaptations of muscular tissue to train-
    ing. Prog Cardiovasc Dis 18:445, 1976

40. Smith JL, Dressendorfer RH, Amsterdam EA: Improved
    exercise tolerance in coronary patients without in-
    creased maximal oxygen uptake (abstract).   Med Sci
    Sports, Spring 1979

41. Clausen JP: Effect of physical training on cardio-
    vascular adjustments to exercise in man.   Physiol
    Rev 57:779, 1977

42. Saltin B: The interplay between peripheral and cen-
    tral factors in the adaptive response to exercise
    and training.   NY Acad Sci 305:224, 1977

9

IN-HOSPITAL REHABILITATION AFTER MYOCARDIAL INFARCTION

Nanette Kass Wenger, M.D.

Introduction

The changing pattern of care for the patient with myocardial infarction in this decade has been characterized by an increase in the early resumption of physical activity and by a consequent decrease in imposed invalidism. Earlier discharge from the hospital is also characteristic for appropriately selected patients, typically on the 10th to 14th day for the patient with an uncomplicated clinical course.

This contrasts markedly with the 1930's advice of Mallory, White, and Salcedo-Salgar: "to advise less than three weeks in bed is unwise, even for patients with the smallest myocardial infarct;" it also contrasts with the statement of Sir Thomas Lewis that "the patient is to be guarded by day and night nursing and helped in every way to avoid voluntary movement or effort."

What We Know

Documentation of the deleterious effects of prolonged immobilization at bed rest has provided the physiologic basis for recommending early mobilization. The most marked of these changes is a decrease in physical work capacity, with as much as a 20 to 25 percent decrement occurring after 3 weeks at bed rest. A decrease of 700 to 800 cc in the circulating blood volume also results from a week to 10 days of strict bed rest. This explains the hypovolemic manifestations of tachycardia and orthostatic hypotension which are observed when the patient

is first mobilized; loss of normal postural vasomotor reflexes potentiates the tachycardia and hypotension. The
hypovolemia, however, imposes an additional problem, in
that the plasma volume decreases to a greater extent
than does the red blood cell mass, increasing blood viscosity and predisposing to thromboembolism; this occurs
in association with decreased use of the leg muscle pump
at bed rest, adding the thromboembolic risk of venous
circulatory stasis to that of increased blood viscosity.

A modest depression of pulmonary ventilation also occurs due to a decrease in lung volume and vital capacity;
negative nitrogen and protein balances are documented,
which may potentially adversely affect myocardial healing; and there is a decrease in skeletal muscle mass and
muscular contractile strength and efficiency; this may
diminish by 10 to 15 percent within the 1st week at bed
rest. Inefficiently contracting muscle demands more oxygen for the same amount of work to be performed, and imposes this increased demand on an impaired oxygen transport system and myocardium.

Three important features of the early ambulation effort are patient selection, program components, and activity surveillance. Patients with uncomplicated myocardial infarction, defined as those without significant
dysrhythmia, heart failure, shock, or persistent or recurrent chest pain, are ideal candidates for early ambulation; such patients constitute almost half of all individuals admitted to coronary care units across the
United States. And, as much as one can generalize about
patients with myocardial infarction, these tend to be
younger patients and patients with an initial episode of
infarction. Patients with complications of myocardial
infarction appear to require management for the specific
problems at bed rest until the complications have been
controlled. Characteristics of early ambulation activities require that they be of low-level intensity,
gradually progressive, and predominantly isotonic in
character. The low-level intensity is generally 1 to 2
mets, one or two times the resting metabolic rate (1 met
= 3.5 cc O_2/kg body weight/min).

These activities generally include self-care, eating,
active and passive arm and leg movement, the use of a
bedside commode, and sitting in bed or in a bedside
chair. Generally accepted criteria for surveillance of
early ambulation involve the avoidance of disproportionate tachycardia, the concept that chest pain, dyspnea,
and/or excessive fatigue should not be precipitated by
activity, the avoidance of dysrhythmias, the avoidance of
increased ST segment displacement on the electrocardiogram or monitor as evidence of ischemia, and the avoidance of systolic hypotension, as the usual response to

140

exercise is a slight increase in systolic blood pressure. Patients whose response to low-level physical activity is appropriate can gradually be progressed to increasing activity loads.

During the remainder of the hospitalization, after discharge from the coronary care unit, early ambulation activities aim to increase function to a level that will enable the post-infarction patient to perform self-care and usual household tasks at the time of discharge from the hospital. Activities are generally of low-level intensity, 2 to 3 mets, and remain primarily isotonic in character. They continue to include active and passive range of motion activities but emphasize walking, gradually increasing the distance and pace of walking.

In recent years, a number of well-designed controlled studies have documented the safety of early ambulation for appropriately selected patients after myocardial infarction. Early ambulation has effected no increase in the hospital complications or in the followup complications of myocardial infarction--angina pectoris, recurrent myocardial infarction, dysrhythmias, congestive heart failure, ventricular aneurysm, cardiac rupture, sudden cardiac death, etc.; indeed, some studies suggested a more favorable outcome. The complications of prolonged immobilization at bed rest--thromboembolism, pulmonary atelectasis, cardiovascular deconditioning, anxiety, and depression--have been effectively reduced. Significantly greater disability (decreased functional capacity) was demonstrated at followup examination with the traditional hospital regimen groups than in the early ambulation groups. The economic advantages are those inherent in a shorter hospitalization and more nearly optimal use of hospital beds and those related to the earlier and more complete return to work of patients in early ambulation programs, probably in conjunction with both physiologic and psychologic rehabilitation components.

What We Must Learn

Information is needed about the detailed effects of early ambulation on myocardial contractility, on myocardial infarction size, and on associated hemodynamic parameters. These studies are now possible with newer and often noninvasive techniques--echocardiography, serial cardiac isoenzyme determinations, myocardial radionuclide studies, etc. The relationship of early exercise stress testing (prior to discharge from the hospital) to early ambulation requires assessment in regard to more precisely defining the effects of early ambulation.

The role of early ambulation for selected subgroups of patients with complicated myocardial infarction must be assessed; does it have added benefit or added risk? Additionally, the various methods and protocols for early ambulation require evaluation to determine an optimal approach to care. For example, we must consider the following questions: Are isometric activities contraindicated in practice, as they are in theory? Should there be increased attention to arm activity? Are different protocols more valuable for the older and younger patients? What is the degree of surveillance necessary, and/or is particular surveillance indicated for certain subgroups of patients? Is there increased value, or, conversely, increased danger of early ambulation in specific subgroups of patients with myocardial infarction? What is the role of early ambulation after myocardial revascularization, identifying both physiologic and psychologic components?

Answers to the above represent the challenge of the 1980's regarding early ambulation.

Bibliography

Benton JG, Brown H, Rusk HA: Energy expended by patients on the bedpan and bedside commode. JAMA 144:1443, 1950

Bloch A, Maeder J-P, Haissly J-C, et al: Early mobilization after myocardial infarction. A controlled study. Am J Cardiol 34:152, 1974

Bonner CD: Rehabilitation instead of bed rest? Geriatrics 24:109, 1969

Boyle JA, Lorimer AR: Early mobilization after uncomplicated myocardial infarction. Prospective study of 538 patients. Lancet 2:346, 1973

Broustet JP, Dubecq M, Bouloumie J, et al: Rehabilitation of the coronary patient: mobilization program in the acute phase. Schweiz Med Wochenschr 103:57, 1973

Chobanian AV, Lille RD, Tercyak A, et al: The metabolic and hemodynamic effects of prolonged bed rest in normal subjects. Circulation 49:551, 1974

Coe WS: Cardiac work and the chair treatment of acute coronary thrombosis. Ann Intern Med 40:42, 1954

DeBusk RF, Spivack AP, van Kessel A, et al: The coronary care unit activities program: its role in post-infarction rehabilitation. J Chron Dis 24:373, 1971

Deitrick JE, Whedon GD, Shorr E: Effects of immobilization upon various metabolic and physiologic functions of
normal men. Am J Med 4:3, 1948

Dock W: The evil sequelae of complete bed rest. JAMA
125:1083, 1944

Duke M: Bed rest in acute myocardial infarction. A
study of physician practices. Am Heart J 82:486, 1971

Fareeduddin K, Abelmann WH: Impaired orthostatic tolerance after bed rest in patients with myocardial infarction. N Engl J Med 280:345, 1969

Groden BM: The management of myocardial infarction. A
controlled study of the effects of early mobilization.
Cardiac Rehabil 1:13, 1971

Groden BM, Brown RIF: Differential psychological effects
of early and late mobilization after myocardial infarction. Scand J Rehabil Med 2:60, 1970

Harpur JE, Kellett RJ, Conner WT, et al: Controlled trial
of early mobilization and discharge from hospital in
uncomplicated myocardial infarction. Lancet 2:1331, 1971

Harrison TR: Abuse of rest as a therapeutic measure of
patients with cardiovascular disease. JAMA 125:1075, 1944

Hayes MJ, Morris GK, Hampton JR: Comparison of mobilization after 2 and 9 days in uncomplicated myocardial
infarction. Br Med J 3:10, 1974

Hutter AM Jr, Sidel VW, Shine KI, et al: Early hospital
discharge after myocardial infarction. N Engl J Med
288:1141, 1973

Hyatt KH, Kamenetsky LG, Smith WM: Extravascular dehydra-
tion as an etiologic factor in post-recumbency orthostat-
ism. Aerosp Med 40:644, 1969

Irvin CW Jr, Burgess AM Jr: The abuse of bed rest in the
treatment of myocardial infarction. N Engl J Med
243:486, 1950

Lamers HJ, Drost WSJ, Kroon BJM, et al: Early mobilization after myocardial infarction: a controlled study.
Br Med J 1:257, 1973

Levine SA: Some harmful effects of recumbency in the
treatment of heart disease. JAMA 126:80, 1944

Lewis T: Diseases of the Heart. New York, Macmillan,
1933, p 49

Lynch TN, Jensen RL, Stevens PM, et al: Metabolic effects of prolonged bed rest: their modification by simulated altitude. Aerosp Med 38:10, 1967

Mallory GK, White PD, Salcedo-Salgar J: The speed of healing of myocardial infarction: a study of the pathologic anatomy in seventy-two cases. Am Heart J 18:647, 1939

McPherson BD, Paivio A, Yuhasz MS, et al: Psychological effects of an exercise program for postinfarct and normal adult men. J Sports Med Phys Fitness 7:95, 1967

Miller PB, Johnson RL, Lamb LE: Effects of moderate physical exercise during four weeks of bed rest on circulatory functions in man. Aerosp Med 36:1077, 1965

Report of the Task Force on Cardiovascular Rehabilitation, National Heart and Lung Institute: Needs and Opportunities for Rehabilitating the Coronary Heart Disease Patient, December 15, 1974. DHEW Publication No (NIH)75-750, Washington DC, 1974

Saltin B, Blomqvist G, Mitchell JH, et al: Response to exercise after bed rest and training. Circulation 37-38 (suppl 7):1, 1968

Swan HJC, Blackburn HW, DeSanctis R, et al: Duration of hospitalization in "uncomplicated acute myocardial infarction." An ad hoc committee review. Am J Cardiol 37:413, 1976

Wanka J: Bedpan vs commode in patients with myocardial infarction. Cardiac Rehabil 1:7, 1970

Wenger NK, Hellerstein HK, Blackburn H, et al: Uncomplicated myocardial infarction. Current physician practice in patient management. JAMA 224:511, 1973

10
POST-HOSPITAL REHABILITATION

Herman K. Hellerstein, M.D.

My assigned objective is to "summarize the state of the
current knowledge and techniques available for the post-
hospital rehabilitation of patients with coronary artery
disease." Of particular interest to the participants in
this workshop is the feasibility and desirability of a
clinical trial for the assessment of physical conditioning and rehabilitation of the cardiac patient.

My comments will reflect a multitude of experiences in
the past 20 years, in large part personal: the Cleveland
Area Heart Association Work Classification Clinic experiences from 1950 to 1963; the earlier nonrandomized Case
Western Reserve University Jewish Community Center Physical Conditioning Program (which spanned the period from
1960 to date with followup data on 252 of 254 subjects);
involvement in the multidisciplinary Report of the Task
Force on Cardiovascular Rehabilitation of the National
Heart and Lung Institute, Needs and Opportunities for
Rehabilitating the Coronary Heart Disease Patient,
December 15, 1974; personal involvement as director of
the Case Western Reserve University Collaborating Center
of the National Exercise and Heart Disease Project; and
familiarity with the published and unpublished experiences of other studies, in Europe (WHO, Sweden, Finland,
Poland) and in Australia and Israel. More detailed information will be presented by several investigators
regarding the latter studies.

In considering exercise conditioning in the rehabilitation of cardiac patients after hospital discharge, it
is essential to consider physical conditioning as a part
of a comprehensive program that involves weight control,
diet therapy, cessation of smoking, regular performance
of prescribed, supervised exercise, continuation of

gainful employment and a normal social mode of life, and adequate recreation and rest.

Rehabilitation has been defined as a process by which the patient is returned realistically to an optimal physiologic, mental-psychological, emotional, sexual, social, vocational, and economic usefulness, and if employable, is provided an opportunity for gainful employment in a competitive world.[1] Physical conditioning through exercise can significantly affect all of the above facets of rehabilitation.

Generally, most patients recover to a moderately successful degree, even without a formal program of rehabilitation.[1] In various studies, more than 80 to 85 percent of employable cardiac patients returned to work, with so-called spontaneous recovery. However, the interval between the discharge from the hospital and return to work may vary from 6 weeks to 6 months or more. This interval between hospital discharge and return to work is determined by many factors: age, social benefits, employment opportunities, past vocational skills and work performance, etc. Dr. Robert Debusk and his associates have suggested that earlier exercise testing and exercise training may shorten this interval, with obvious economic implications.

Our experiences at the Cleveland Work Classification Clinic indicated that 80 to 85 percent of myocardial infarct patients with employment problems could also resume working. It became clear that patients with coronary disease could work productively in a great variety of gainful occupations, without hazard to themselves, fellow workers, and employees.[2] Many of the jobs required the expenditure of relatively high energy levels.[3] The success in returning to the world of work is one of the simplest ways of assessing the results and clinical value of medical care, and particularly of physical conditioning if the work requirements are significant, i.e., about 4 to 5 MET's. (An MET is defined as the oxygen uptake/kg bw min sitting quietly in a chair or at supine rest. Generally, this represents 3.5 to 4.0 ml of O_2/kg bw X min.)

The earlier activation in ambulation, now accepted as part of an in-hospital rehabilitation program, has been responsible in large part for the decreased post-hospital discharge occurrence of weakness, depression, anxiety, and low self-esteem, etc.[4]

In the last two decades, numerous exercise training programs for post-myocardial infarction patients have developed, and their supervisors have reported remarkably consistent improvement in cardiovascular function in 75 to 85 percent of the subjects, despite great differences

146

in the design of the studies, supervision, monitoring, and methods of assessment.[5] The similarities of the beneficial effects outweigh the differences.

Assessment of Results of Training

The effects of physical conditioning have been assessed clinically and from the standpoints of cardiovascular function; hormonal changes; body specific gravity; psychological, emotional, and vocational changes; sexual activity; morbidity; mortality; and the "quality of living."

The clinical assessment of value of physical conditioning programs has included changes in lifestyle, changes in frequency and quality of sexual activity, recording of hospitalizations, changes in medication requirements, intercurrent hospitalizations, illnesses, recurrent infarction, coronary surgery, and mortality.

The cardiovascular effects include changes of peak performance; occasionally measured maximal oxygen uptake; decreased tension time index; variable effects on stroke volume, ejection fraction, dP/dt, and left ventricular end-diastolic pressure; reduction of hypertensive blood pressure values in exercise; decrease of peripheral resistance, of the heart rate at rest, during sleep, during sexual activity, and during effort; electrocardiographic changes including quantitative lessening of ST segment displacement; variable effects on ventricular ectopic activity; and enhanced oxygen extraction by the peripheral skeletal muscle tissues.[6]

Visualization of the coronary artery anatomy by cardiac catheterization and angiograms showed that enhancement of intercoronary collaterals was rarely demonstrated after physical training of coronary subjects.[7] An increase in coronary intercoronary collaterals was generally associated with progressive stenosis of one or more coronary arteries. Only an occasional report has appeared on changes in the endocardial and subepicardial distribution after training.[8] Ventricular fibrillation occurring in supervised monitored training areas has been uncommon and with rare exception has been reversible, almost always with complete recovery.

Metabolic and hormonal responses are reflected by decreased lactate production for the same workload, lowering of serum catecholamines and of serum lipid levels (especially in Type IV hyperlipoproteinemia), an increased ratio of high density lipoprotein-cholesterol (HDL-C) to total cholesterol, reduction of adipose tissue

147

and an increase of lean body mass, reduction of serum insulin level and insulin glucagon ratio, changes in blood clotting and fibrinolysis.[5]

Psychological changes include an improvement of subjective well-being and decrease of depression, family adjustments and attitudes, and enhancement of the quality and frequency of sexual activity. The vocational effects were assessed by the success in the return to work, and performance and adjustment at work.

These effects have influenced favorably the "quality of living." The major prospective randomized, supervised, and monitored programs of physical conditioning of coronary subjects (NEHDP and the WHO European Study) have not yet reported the effect on recurrence of infarction, or on mortality. Other studies, plagued by significant noncompliance, drop-ins, and other programmatic difficulties, suggest that such participation conferred little protection from morbidity or mortality.

From the above, it is obvious that involvement in an exercise training program involved more than changes in the cardiovascular system.

Techniques of Exercise Testing
and Assessment of Responses

Considerable progress has been made in methods for quantitative exercise testing, quantitative exercise prescription, and quantitative exercise training. The comparability of the responses to exercise testing of the lower extremities has been demonstrated for testing by bicycle ergometer, treadmill, or steps. The assessment of the effects of exercise training can now be expressed quantitatively in terms of the chronotropic, aerobic, and myocardial aerobic capacities and changes in electrical functions.[8] They have been found to be useful in evaluating functions and responses to various types of interventions (i.e., not only physical conditioning but also drug therapy and surgery). It is beyond the scope of this presentation to detail the methods of assessment of chronotropic reserve and impairment, aerobic capacity and impairment, and myocardial aerobic capacity (which is dependent upon the excellent correlation between measured myocardial oxygen uptake and two of its major determinants, heart rate and systolic blood pressure). It is probable that Dr. Robert Bruce has presented this in greater detail.

The primary objective of exercise testing of post-infarction patients is not the establishment of the diagnosis of coronary disease, but rather to evaluate quantitatively cardiovascular functions, i.e., changes in chronotropic, aerobic, myocardial aerobic, and electrical parameters.

With the advent of quantitative exercise electrocardiography, particularly by on-line computer analysis, a new dimension (time) has been added to the testing of cardiac electrical functions.

New insight has been obtained in the importance of ST-T segment displacement in coronary patients.[6] Exercise ST-T segment responses have greater value when quantitated and related to the development of symptoms, the level of effort at which they occur, and the duration of their persistence after completion of the exercise test. An increase in ST displacement at low work levels and of low heart rate and blood pressure and their product is consistent with deterioration of cardiovascular functions.

Although there is a generally good relationship between structure and function, paradoxically there can be discordance in the impairments. For example, it has been shown that subjects with coronary disease who had excellent aerobic capacity, chronotropic myocardial VO_2 capacity, still developed asymptomatic marked ischemic ST changes at relatively low levels of work and heart rate.

Techniques of electrocardiographic recording improved the yield of abnormal responses to exercise. Recently there has been awareness that multiple leads reflecting at least X, Y, and Z components of the electrocardiogram are necessary in order to enhance the sensitivity of the exercise response. The use of a single unipolar or bipolar V5 lead is associated with a large number (approximately 11 percent) of false negative (normal) responses.[6]

Techniques of Exercise Prescription

There is general agreement that exercise testing is a prerequisite for exercise prescription.[6] In general, considerable insight has been gained into the importance of the various factors which modify the exercise prescription, i.e., age, sex, health status, current medication, orthopedic and musculoskeletal integrity, degree of motivation, individual recreational preferences, and most importantly, the diagnostic and functional evaluation obtained from exercise tests. There is general agreement that exercise sessions should include a warm-up period, endurance phase, and a cool-down period. The endurance phase should be prescribed in terms of intensity, duration, frequency, and type of activity. In assessing results of physical conditioning programs, it is essential to have firm documentation of compliance: attendance at exercise sessions and quantitative measures of the intensity as well as frequency and duration.

An approximation of the intensity of effort has been made in general from the well-established relationship between the peak attained heart rate and the peak oxygen uptake. Generally, both in normals and cardiacs, 70 to 85 percent of the peak attained heart rate corresponds to approximately 60 to 78 percent of peak oxygen uptake.[9] Recording of the average and peak heart rate during training sessions provides some objective evidence that the individual has exercised in a range which generally indicates that the aerobic metabolism is being stressed. At this relative range, several key physiologic and biochemical changes can transpire which indicate that the individual's aerobic metabolism is being stressed: the respiratory exchange ratio approaches unity; there are increases in blood lactic acid, fibrinolytic activity, urinary catecholamine excretion, capacity to oxidize fatty acids, the release of fatty acids from adipose tissues, the capacity to regenerate ATP by oxidative phosphorylation, increased protein content of mitochondrial fraction of skeletal muscle, etc.

These are desirable changes. However, in practical experience many patients do not attain the desired heart rate because of ventricular ectopic activity occurring before the desired heart rate, cardiac symptoms, skeletal muscle difficulties, etc. The method of recording the heart rate and arrhythmias during every exercise session entails considerable equipment, data monitoring, and recording. There is a need for a simpler method to assess the intensity (energy expenditure) and some measure of myocardial oxygen uptake during training. Such methods are presently not feasible on a mass scale.

Unimpressive responses to training programs may be due to inadequate intensity. The successful and safe high level exercise testing of cardiac patients has emboldened investigators to increase the intensity of training. The result has been a significant augmentation of improvement in aerobic capacity. For example, in the early 1960 to 1968 Cleveland Jewish Community Center studies, the oxygen uptake increased from 24.7 to 29.2 ml O_2/kg bw/min. Approximately a decade later,[10] similar ASHD subjects trained at a more intense level, and the maximal oxygen uptake increased from 24.9 to 34.8 ml O_2/kg bw/min, which represented an increase of functional aerobic capacity from 62 to 95 percent, in contrast to the early experience of 62 to 78 percent functional aerobic capacity.

While the optimal intensive exercise is thought to be within the range of 60 to 70 percent of the VO_2 maximaximum, training at considerably lower levels has been found, surprisingly, to produce significant improvements in the VO_2 max.[9] In the pre-randomization phase of the National Exercise and Heart Disease Project, significant improvement transpired when subjects were trained at a considerably lower level. As a matter of fact, this improvement complicated interpretation of the effects of exercise training in the post-randomized period.

Training specificity

In the assessment of results of physical conditioning, it is important to incorporate in training programs a recognition of training specificity.[6] Numerous investigations have shown that cardiorespiratory training responses are best demonstrated when the subjects is due to local adaptation in the skeletal muscle trained. For example, swim training or one-leg training does not improve the running VO_2 maximum. Similar findings were reported by Clausen between two groups of men. One group exercised using their arms and the other using their legs. In the tests after training, both groups alternated between arm and leg exercise, using the same exercise protocol. Training of arm muscles affected heart rate responses only during arm exercise and vice versa.

Implications of training specificity

The lack of significant cardiovascular crossover benefits of training of upper extremity and lower extremity and vice versa implies that a substantial portion of the conditioning effects are derived from increased peripheral AV oxygen extraction by exercising muscle. Training specificity has significant implication for design of cardiac exercise training programs. Since few recreational and occupational activities require sustained lower extremity exertion, the rationale of the prevalent practice of restricting exercise training to lower extremities appears questionable.

The principle of specificity of training has largely been ignored in the planning of most adult fitness cardiac exercise training programs. Many cardiac reconditioning programs--with the exception of the ongoing National Exercise and Heart Disease Project--are based on lower extremity training by walking, jogging, or stationary bicycling. Such programs are limited in scope, ignore the group of patients who--because of orthopedic problems, arthritis, or peripheral vascular disease--have significant limitation in performance of lower extremity

activities, and furthermore neglect to consider daily
living activities which employ all major muscle groups.
In individuals whose occupations require arm movements
there is a need to be concerned with training of these
muscle groups.

Techniques to Assess Mechanisms of Benefits

The beneficial effects of exercise conditioning have
been easier to identify and to quantitate than to explain. The local changes in the peripheral skeletal
musculature readily account for the increased AV oxygen
extraction. The myocardium in humans has not been shown
to develop an increase of myofibrillar ATPase as it does
in the rat but not in the dog.[11] However, the reduction
in plasma epinephrine and norepinephrine at rest and after peak effort and of myocardial epinephrine uptake may
account for the reduced heart rate and blood pressure
after physical and sexual effort and the decreased myocardial oxygen requirements for a given workload. Several studies have shown no increase of intercoronary
collaterals or reversal of atherosclerosis by physical
training.[7]

The exact mechanisms by which physical conditioning
affects cardiac patients remain uncertain. In part,
this is because of the predominant clinical and "nonbasic
science" orientation of most of the earlier investigations and in large part because of the deficiencies of
the available techniques at the time studies were begun
some 20 years ago.

The mechanism by which significant improvement in cardiovascular functions transpired needs clarification.
For example, are there changes in the neurohormonal receptors (adrenergic, muscarinic serotoninergic) in the
central nervous system, and particularly the location in
the heart (in the endocardium and/or subepicardium area),
or in the peripheral musculature and vasculature system?
The changes in cardiovascular functions have not been
adequately characterized sufficiently to explain the improvement of function even in the presence of significant
multivessel coronary disease. The changes in catecholamines in the serum and myocardial uptake provide an important lead.[11]

How are these related to the biogenic amines, endor-
phins, etc., to mood, and to emotional and psychological
responses? The changes in psychological mood, self-
esteem, etc., have not been explained on a biochemical
basis, nor has insight been provided as to what parts of
the nervous system are involved. The improvement in mood

152

and emotion may be the result of the summation of the metabolic and cardiovascular changes, in large part due to restoration of physical strength, cardiovascular reserve, sexual performance, and self-esteem. Insight is needed to explain the depression which is one of the most common complications of myocardial infarction and the relatively good outlook for rehabilitation of subjects who use denial rather than depression in reacting to their illness.[12]

What are the mechanisms by which certain characteristics of physical training (especially the intensity at given levels of the aerobic capacity) trigger significant adaptation in a multitude of systems (metabolic, oxidative, clotting, etc.)? Can this be duplicated by non-exercise methods--for example, dobutamine infusions, meditation, relaxation, etc.?

The coronary arterial circulation tree (and the coronary distribution regional and laminar, blood flow, myocardial perfusion, myocardial metabolism, ventricular functions, etc.) need clarification. The nonisotopic assessment of cardiac output, systolic time intervals, and noninvasive nonisotopic methods merit further application to clarify these unanswered questions.

Factors Influencing Response to Training Programs

Failure to respond to a physical conditioning program depends not only on the design, costs, availability, management, acceptance, motivation, compliance, and adherence, but even more importantly on the primary determinant, namely, the severity of the underlying disease process. Patients who are unable to perform at least 2 or 3 MET's are generally ineligible for participation in exercise training programs. However, this represents only 3 to 4 percent of all myocardial infarct patients. Patients with poor rehabilitation potential often show severely reduced inotropic and/or chronotropic reserve, severe angina pectoris, myocardial dyskinesia and/or aneurysm, frequent ventricular ectopic arrhythmias or pronounced ST segment displacement during or after exercise.

Our previously published experience indicates that approximately 15 percent of postmyocardial infarction patients showed minimal or no improvement despite faithful attendance and active participation in an exercise program.[13] Coronary arteriograms demonstrated severe involvement of three major arteries and stenosis of 90 percent or greater of two major arteries. Thus the severity and progression of the underlying coronary disease represents a major obstacle to improvement. The development of myocardial imaging techniques, and hopefully development of noncatheterization demonstration of the coronary artery circulation in all patients to be considered for physical conditioning, would identify those who would not benefit immediately from a physical conditioning program and would probably be eligible for other medical or surgical intervention. For this reason, coronary arteriograms and myocardial imaging during multistage exercise testing should be seriously recommended to exclude patients unlikely to profit from a conditioning program.

These studies would supplement clinical observations and indirect assessment of the severity of coronary disease by the level of the maximal aerobic capacity, blood pressure responses (failure to increase blood pressure during effort), changes in arrhythmias, ST displacement, systolic time intervals, etc.

Epicrisis

Unresolved questions and future challenges

Despite the substantial attainments cited above, there are many needs and deficiencies in regard to training (methodology, effectiveness, facilities, and cost), research, and societal applications.

Training

There is a need to determine optimal intensity of training and the number of years to demonstrate substantial long-term training effects, to enhance adherence to training programs by identifying susceptible dropouts, to avoid the danger of "therapeutic nihilism," to reduce the economic cost, and to determine the cost-effectiveness of various rehabilitation procedures.

Research

There is a need for better understanding of the adaptation of individuals to intervention at the cellular, organ, and individual levels; for evaluation of methods of exercise testing and training and their relationship to specific occupations; for more research on the impact of illness and of health maintenance on society at large; and for more basic research on the pathogenic factors of heart disease and especially on the progression of arteriosclerosis before and after myocardial infarction.

The rehabilitation programs must include patient education, selection of appropriate therapy, and societal involvement.

To determine whether rehabilitation efforts enhance the length as well as the quality of life, it is necessary to have the results of prospectively large scale randomized studies, not only for the coronary prone, but also for subjects with infarction and postcoronary surgery. There is need for a sufficient number of subjects (not found in the Canadian, USA NEHDP, or European WHO studies), and for variations in the design of exercise training to determine whether long-range adherence is feasible at reasonable cost. There is a need to improve practical and optimal types of rehabilitation facilities and to determine the value of physical conditioning as a valid rehabilitation measure after coronary and noncoronary surgery.

As stated elsewhere, technologies and methodologies which are available at a given time determine in large part the questions which can be asked and the directions of further investigations.[14] With the blossoming field of receptor sites, biochemistry of the brain, noninvasive myocardial characterization imaging, etc., it is possible to ask cogent new questions.

We are, I hope, at the dawn of a scientific era which will incorporate rehabilitation with basic sciences.[11] We may expect many new discoveries relevant to rehabilitation and to physical conditioning, due to an interplay of information about nutrition, behavior, physiology, psychology, and health maintenance. It is easy to point to new scientific techniques, such as CT scanning, which Dr. Wood in Minnesota is developing, and other noninvasive devices, which--if used in the next few years--will make it possible to characterize the coronary circulation and the myocardial function. These and other technologic advances may not be the only factors. The great periods of discovery in science are marked by the sudden synthesis of knowledge from different fields seemingly as dissimilar as chemistry, sociology, economics, communications, behavioral theory, and interscience.[14] This, then, is a challenge facing the National Institutes of Health.

References

1. Rehabilitation of Patients with Cardiovascular Disease. Report of a WHO Committee. World Health Organization, Technical Report Series No. 270, Geneva, 1964

2. Parran TV, Hellerstein HK, Cohen D, Goldston E: Results of studies at the work classification clinic of the Cleveland Area Heart Society. In, Work and the Heart (Rosenbaum FF, Belknap EL, eds). New York, Hoeber, 1959, chap 38, p 330

3. Hellerstein HK: Prescription of vocational and leisure activities. Practical aspects. In, Advances in Cardiology (Konig K, ed). S Karger AG, Basel, Switzerland, 24:56, 1978

4. Wenger NK, Hellerstein HK: (eds). Rehabilitation of the Coronary Patient. New York, John Wiley, 1978

5. Naughton JP, Hellerstein HK: (eds). Exercise Testing and Exercise Training in Coronary Heart Disease. New York, Academic Press, 1973

6. Hellerstein HK, Franklin BA: Exercise testing and prescription. In, Rehabilitation of the Coronary Patient, (Wenger NK, Hellerstein HK, eds). New York, John Wiley, 1978, p 149

7. Hellerstein HK: A misguided goal or unrealized objective. Panel V: acceleration of collaterals due to physical activity--dogma or fact. In, Critical Evaluation of Cardiac Rehabilitation, (Kellerman JJ, Denolin H, eds). S Karger AG, Basel, Switzerland 1977, p 125

8. Bove AA, Hultgren PB, Ritzer TF, Carey RA: Myocardial blood flow and hemodynamic responses to exercise training in dogs. J Appl Physiol 46(3):571, 1979

9. Hellerstein HK, Hirsch EZ, Ader R, Greenblott N, Siegel M: Principles of exercise prescription. Normals and cardiac subjects. In, Exercise Testing and Exercise Training in Coronary Heart Disease (Naughton JP, Hellerstein HK, eds). New York, Academic Press, 1973, p 129

10. Hellerstein HK: Limitations of marathon running in the rehabilitation of coronary patients. Anatomic and physiologic determinants. In, The Marathon: Physiological, Medical, Epidemiological and Psychological Studies (Milvey P, ed). Ann NY Acad Sci 301:484, 1977

11. Hellerstein HK: Rehabilitation of the post-infarction patient. In, Diagnosis and Therapy of Coronary Artery Disease (Cohn Peter F, ed). Little Brown & Co, 1979

12. Stern MJ, Pascale L, McLoone JB: Psychosocial adap-
    tation following an acute myocardial infaction. J
    Chron Dis 29:513, 1976

13. Hellerstein HK: Anatomic factors influencing ef-
    fects of exercise therapy of ASHD subjects (Roskamm
    H, Reindell H, eds). In, Das Chronisch Kranke Herz.
    New York, FK Schattauer Verlag-Stuttgart, 1973, p
    513

14. Hellerstein HK, Katz LN: Electrocardiography. In,
    Circulation of the Blood. Men and Ideas (Fishman
    AP, Richards DW, eds). New York, Oxford Press,
    1964, Vol 5, p 265

11

CARDIOVASCULAR COMPLICATIONS DURING MEDICALLY SUPERVISED EXERCISE TRAINING

William L. Haskell, Ph.D.

Comprehensive programs of cardiac rehabilitation frequently include a program of increased physical activity. The major reasons usually cited for encouraging
cardiac patients to exercise include enhancement of cardiovascular function, improvement of psychological status
and a reduction in new clinical manifestations including
angina pectoris, cardiac arrest, and myocardial infarction. These exercise recommendations are made even
though the specific benefits derived from an increase in
physical activity by cardiac patients have not been fully
established nor has the relative safety of such participation been defined.

Patient safety is an important consideration in the
use of exercise training for the reconditioning of the
cardiac patient. The fact that exercise, by increasing
myocardial work, can precipitate a sudden discrepancy between myocardial oxygen supply and demand--which in turn
can trigger cardiac arrest or myocardial infarction in
coronary artery disease patients--is generally accepted.
When designing an activity plan for cardiac patients, the
safety of a particular approach appears closely related
to successfully identifying and excluding patients with
ventricular dysfunction or electrical instability at rest
or during even mild exercise and prescribing for appropriate patients an activity regimen which maintains them
well within their exercise tolerance.

Even with such precautions during patient evaluation
and development of an exercise prescription, patients do
develop major cardiovascular complications, even during
medically supervised exercise programs. This presentation reviews information regarding the frequency of such
complications, factors associated with their occurrence,

and research needed to help increase the safety of exercise training when performed by cardiac patients.

Early Reports of Complications

Early reports regarding cardiovascular complications during exercise by cardiac patients focused on individual incidences of cardiac arrest or myocardial infarction[1,2] or the occurrence of these events in separate exercise programs during their initial years of operation.[3,4,5] These reports, while valuable in demonstrating the need for safety considerations, including the value of electrical defibrillation, did not provide data on the rate of complications to be expected during exercise training nor information on patient selection or characteristics of program design which might lead to improved patient safety.

Several of the earlier reports indicated that serious cardiovascular complications, especially cardiac arrest, can be a reasonably common event during medically supervised cardiac exercise programs,[5,6] while no such complications have been reported by others.[7,8] In an attempt to obtain some indication of both the frequency and nature of major cardiovascular complications during individually prescribed and medically supervised exercise programs, a retrospective survey of selected cardiac exercise programs was conducted in the United States and Canada from 1974 to 1976.[9]

Survey of Cardiac Exercise Programs in the United States and Canada

A brief questionnaire was mailed to directors of exercise programs that met predetermined criteria regarding their design and method of operation. To be included in the survey, each exercise program had to meet the following minimal criteria, specifying that: (1) the exercise program be designed and operated specifically for cardiac patients, (2) a medical examination be required on entry and at least annually thereafter, (3) all exercise sessions be medically supervised with the capability to provide cardiopulmonary resuscitation including emergency medications and electrical defibrillation, and (4) the program had been in operation for at least one year. No program was excluded from the survey if it met these criteria.

The questionnaire was designed to elicit information regarding the starting date of the program, the number of cardiac patients who had participated since the inception of the program, the number and type of nonfatal or fatal cardiovascular complications occurring while patients were involved in an exercise session or any time proximal to the exercise session which might be interpreted as resulting from their participation, criteria for patient entry (i.e., patient medical status, weeks postinfarction, etc.), number of exercise sessions per week, characteristics of the exercise training program, and the type and extent of medical supervision provided during the exercise training sessions. When a questionnaire was not returned, a second questionnaire was sent, which was then followed by a telephone call or personal contact in order to obtain information from all programs surveyed.

Results

Questionnaires were sent to the directors of 30 programs and results were obtained from each one for a 100 percent response rate. Data from a majority of these programs still operational in January 1977 were updated by repeat questionnaires, so that the results of the survey would include recent experience as well as experience obtained as early as 1960-65 for several programs.

The 30 programs participating in the survey represented 103 exercise class locations in North America. These classes were conducted in several different types of exercise facilities; 21 were located in YMCA's or YMHA's, 45 in hospitals, 11 in universities, and 26 in independent facilities such as medical clinics or office buildings. Fourteen of the 30 programs (44 percent) bebegan before 1970, with 11 of these 14 still in operation in January 1977, while only one of the 16 initiated since 1970 was no longer operating.

The minimum time following myocardial infarction or cardiac surgery before a patient was allowed into an exercise program ranged from 2 to 12 weeks, with a median of 8 weeks and a mean of 9 weeks. The number of exercise sessions recommended per week ranged from one to five, with a mean and median of three sessions per week. The most prevalent forms of exercise were walking, jogging, running, and calisthenics, with approximately one-half (17 of 30) of the programs including some type of active games.

All programs provided on-site medical supervision of the exercise sessions. Supervision was provided primarily by physicians, but an increasing number of the newer programs reported using cardiovascular (CCU) trained nurses. Medical supervision in 28 of the programs included checking with patients who had medically related questions at the beginning of or during an exercise session, examining or recording the ECG or blood pressure of patients whose disease status possibly had changed since their most recent training session, providing instruction on related topics, and the providing of medical care in the case of an emergency. In the two other programs, additional medical supervision was provided by continuous ECG monitoring performed by specially trained cardiovascular nurses during each exercise session. In these two programs, subjects exercised on stationary bicycles, motor driven treadmills, or rowing machines while their electrocardiograms were monitored using telemetry or hardware recording equipment including oscilloscopes and strip chart recorders.

Number of Patients

During the period surveyed, 13,570 patients were reported enrolled in the 30 programs, and they contributed to a total of 1,629,634 patient-hours of exercise participation. It is estimated that each time a patient participated in an exercise session he was at the exercise facility approximately 1 hour. Thus, if a patient participated in a program 3 times per week for 30 weeks he contributed 90 patient-hours to the total, or if a class of 30 patients met 3 times per week that would be 90 patient-hours of participation. The average number of exercise sessions participated in by each patient was 111, or the equivalent of 37 weeks of participation 3 times per week.

Cardiovascular Complications

During the 1,629,634 hours of participation, a total of 61 major cardiovascular complications was reported. These complications were recorded as cardiac arrest, myocardial infarction, or other, and as fatal or nonfatal. The distribution of the 60 events among these categories is provided in table 1. Fourteen events were fatal, while 47 nonfatal cardiac arrests or myocardial infarctions were reported. Of the 50 cardiac arrests, 42 (84 percent) were successfully resuscitated and 8 (16 percent) were fatal, while 5 (71 percent) of the 7 patients with documented myocardial infarction recovered. Four other fatal complications included two attributed to

162

pulmonary embolism and one each as a result of pulmonary edema and cardiogenic shock. These four deaths occurred following exercise sessions, during which symptoms developed and the patient was hospitalized.

Table 1: Major Cardiovascular Complications During Exercise Training of Cardiac Patients

	Nonfatal	Fatal	Total
Cardiac arrest	42* (38,801)†	8 (203,704)	50 (32,593)
Myocardial infarction	5 (325,927)	2 (814,816)	7 (232,805)
Other	--	4 (407,408)	4 (407,408)
TOTAL	47 (34,673)	14 (116,402)	61 (26,715)

*Number of events for each classification.

†Number of patient-hours of participation per event--average for all 30 programs surveys, with a total of 1,629,634 patient-hours of participation.

An attempt was made to determine the frequency of nonfatal complications other than cardiac arrest or myocardial infarction, but because of the extremely variable recordkeeping and reporting rate by the different programs, these data were not included in the analyses.

Complication Rate

By dividing the patient-hours of participation by the number of complications, a complication rate expressed as the number of patient-hours per event for each category was obtained. The mean complication rates for the 30 programs surveyed for nonfatal cardiac arrest and myocardial infarction and for fatal cardiac arrest, myocardial infarction, and other causes are provided in table 1. Cardiac arrest was by far the most frequent complication, with a rate of one event per 32,593 patient-hours (nonfatal plus fatal), while myocardial infarction on the average was reported only once every 232,809 patient-hours. The overall rate for all complications recorded (fatal and nonfatal) was one event every 26,715 patient-hours. The fatal complication rate was one mortality every 116,402 patient-hours of participation.

The two programs that included continuous electrocardiographic monitoring of all patients during exercise training sessions reported a total of three nonfatal cardiac arrests during a total of 352,200 patient-hours of experience for a complication rate of one event per 117,333 participant-hours. This experience was accumulated from a total of 3,940 patients participating at 70 exercise class locations in the United States between 1970 and 1976. The experience for the 28 programs that did not conduct continuous ECG monitoring during exercise training was one major complication (fatal or nonfatal) every 22,028 patient-hours. The difference in these two rates is significant at P <0.01.

Based on information collected during this survey, the difference in complication rates reported by programs during 1970-1976 cannot be explained readily by how soon patients enter a program after hospitalization, by the type of exercise performed (walking, jogging, games, or calisthenics), or by the type of facility in which the program is operated (i.e., YMCA vs. hospital). Some of the differences in event rates may be due to differences in the characteristics of the warming-up or tapering-off periods at the beginning and end of the class, respectively, since these are the times when the greatest number of complications appear to develop, especially cardiac arrest. Of the 61 complications reported in table 1, at least 44 occurred either during the warm-up phase or during the cool-down or tapering-off period at the end of the exercise session. It is not possible to determine from this survey if the complication rate is related to the intensity of exercise performed during the session.

The one program characteristic which appears to influence the cardiovascular complication rate, especially the fatal complication rate, is the use of continuous electrocardiographic (ECG) monitoring during the exercise training session. Even though both the nonfatal and fatal complication rates are significantly lower in the two ECG monitored programs as compared to the rates for 28 programs not using continuous monitoring, some of this difference might be due to other program characteristics.

For example, the patient-to-medical supervisor ratio ranges from 1-to-1 to 4-to-1 in the continually monitored programs, while in the group supervised programs it typically ranges from 10-to-1 up to 35-to-1. Just this closer medical supervision, without continuous ECG monitoring, might result in greater patient safety by identifying changes in patient symptoms prior to the occurrence of a major cardiovascular complication, thus preventing the complication from developing. Also, closer supervision might help prevent patients from exercising above their prescribed intensity and eliciting myocardial ischemia or electrical instability.

164

Recent Reduction in Complication Rate

As stated in the previous section, when the mortality rate for all cardiac exercise programs is expressed as the number of deaths per participant-hours of exposure, the rate is 1 death every 116,402 participant-hours. However, if the mortality rate is calculated only for those programs operating in 1976 that had been in operation for at least 1 year at that time, the rate changes to one death every 212,182 participant-hours (p <.001).

The Cardio Pulmonary Research Institute in Seattle, Washington, has been conducting exercise training programs since 1968. During this time the Institute has accumulated a total of 260,254 participant-hours of exercise training with 23 nonfatal complications for a nonfatal complication rate of one event every 11,315 participant-hours (no in-class fatalities have occurred). From 1968 to 1975, during which time there were 16 cardiac arrests and 3 myocardial infarctions in 150,580 participant-hours of experience, the complication rate was 1 nonfatal event every 7,925 participant-hours. In contrast to this earlier experience, since 1975 there have been only 4 nonfatal cardiac arrests in 109,674 participant-hours of experience, for an event rate of 1 per 27,418 participant-hours (see table 2).

Table 2: Recent vs. Earlier Complications Rate in CAPRI Cardiac Exercise Program

Event	1968 - 1975	1975 - 1979	1968 - 1979
Cardiac arrest	16	4	20
Myocardial infarction	3	0	3
TOTAL	19	4	23
Participant-hours	150,580	109,674	260,254
Event rate	1/7,925	1/27,418	1/11,315

Experience reported to April 1979: all nonfatal events.

Research Directed at Increasing Safety of Exercise Training by Cardiac Patients

The safety of exercise training by cardiac patients might be enhanced by investigating the following questions.

1. Can prognostic criteria be developed to better identify those patients at highest risk of exertion-induced cardiac arrest? Current criteria allow for identification of patients at very high risk of recurrent manifestations (at rest as well as exercise) but not those patients currently considered eligible for exercise training. Can criteria be developed that will not result in excessive false positives (patients excluded from exercise training for whom it would be safe) as well as false negatives?

2. Can objective criteria be developed for determining the appropriate level of medical supervision required during exercise training of cardiac patients classified by clinical and/or functional status?

3. What are the appropriate criteria to use in determining the eligibility of a cardiac patient to graduate from a medically supervised exercise program to a non-supervised program?

4. Can new, easy-to-use, and relatively inexpensive monitoring equipment and delivery systems be developed to aid in the detection of significant changes in electrical stability of the myocardium that would be prognostic for exertion-induced or related cardiac arrest?

5. What level of medical supervision (physician, nurse, paramedic, etc.) of cardiac exercise programs is required to insure patient safety? What criteria should be used to graduate patients to programs providing less intense and less costly supervision?

6. What criteria should be used in promoting unsupervised exercise training programs for cardiac patients who do not have ready access to a supervised program? Can stationary exercise equipment and telephone transmission of the ECG be used to guide such programs during the early phase of recovery?

References

1. Naughton J, Bruhn J, Letegola MT: Rehabilitation following myocardial infarction. Am J Med 46:725, 1969

2. Pyfer H, Doane BL: Cardiac arrest during exercise training. JAMA 210: 101, 1969

3. Cantwell JD, Fletcher GF: Cardiac complications while jogging. JAMA 210:130, 1969

4. Pyfer H, Doane B, Mead W, Frederick R: Group exercise rehabilitation for cardiopulmonary patients. Med Sci Sports 5:71, 1973

5. Hakkila J: Complications during physical rehabilitation of coronary patients. G Ital Cardiol 3:632, 1973

6. Mead WF, Pyfer HR, Trombold JC, Frederick RC: Successful resuscitation of near simultaneous cases of cardiac arrest with a review of fifteen cases occurring during supervised exercise. Circulation 53:187, 1976

7. Sanne H: Exercise tolerance and physcial training of non-selected patients after myocardial infarction. Acta Med Scand (suppl) 551:1, 1973

8. Kentala E: Physical fitness and feasibility of physical rehabilitation after myocardial infarction in men of working age. Ann Clin Res (suppl) 9:1, 1972

9. Haskell WL: Cardiovascular complications of exercise training by cardiac patients. Circulation 57:920, 1978

SUMMARY: PART 3

John Naughton, M.D.

Dr. Henry Taylor reviewed the status of studies performed on presumably healthy middle-aged adults. Although more than 50 such studies have been reported during the past quarter century, none provides conclusive evidence of the value of chronic physical activity as a primary preventer of the clinical manifestations of coronary heart disease, especially death. Despite this circumstance there is sufficient evidence which suggests that physical activity acts as a deterrent to clinically manifest CHD. The question seems to be, "Does physical activity exert a protective effect which can be masked or overwhelmed when other risk factors are present in high concentration?" Clearly, data obtained by Keys and Taylor and later reviewed by Leon and Blackburn suggest that form and substance may be important determinants of the role of physical activity. In other words, the performance of activity on a regular basis may be important, and a daily energy expenditure in excess of 350 kcal per day may be required to insure the desired protection.

Dr. Taylor is convinced that physical activity requires definitive investigation. He suggests that it is easier to study physical inactivity than physical activity. Since he is convinced that it is inordinately expensive and impractical to mount a primary intervention study, Dr. Taylor strongly supports the concept that the effects of physical activity on myocardial infarction subjects be studied. If a properly mounted and conducted trial of secondary intervention were conducted, he would be satisfied that its results could be translated to primary intervention. He argues for a unifactorial rather than multifactorial study so that the issue of the effects of physical activity on CHD could be resolved once and for all.

Dr. Ezra Amsterdam presented his observations on CHD subjects treated with coronary artery bypass surgery who were subjected to later physical activity intervention. His observations indicate that cardiovascular adaptation to submaximal exercise stress is enhanced by surgical treatment. However, myocardial performance may still be inadequate. Addition of regular physical activity after recovering from surgical intervention may offer this group of CHD patients an even more favorable long-term outlook. His findings clearly suggest a need for studies designed to delineate the effects of physical conditioning on central cardiovascular mechanisms as compared to peripheral vascular and musculoskeletal mechanisms.

Dr. Herman Hellerstein reviewed the history of cardiac rehabilitation, with which he has been so intimately associated. He seemed to question the value of clinical trials, based on his concern about patient selection. Furthermore, he seemed to question the potential value of a single intervention therapy for a multifactoral disease, and emphasized the importance of central nervous system factors in the pathogenesis of CHD.

Dr. Nanette Kass Wenger reviewed the history of early ambulation postmyocardial infarction. Her presentation emphasized the benefits of preventing unnecessary physical deconditioning, the psychological benefits of early ambulation, and the importance of patient-spouse education. She seemed to propose a need for studies of early post-MI exercise testing, but did not come off as an outspoken convenient proponent of this approach as a means of evaluating post-MI functional status or of identifying high risk and low risk CHD survivors.

Dr. William Haskell reviewed his, Dr. Blackburn's, and Dr. Wenger's efforts to identify the risks associated with physical activity programs for post-MI patients. Although their data were clearly retrospective and subject to the pitfalls and criticisms associated with questionnaire surveys, it was apparent that the investigators had a good response rate and the data were analyzed critically. They identified a risk rate of 61 fatal and nonfatal complications for every 26,715 hours of formal physical activity. Cardiac arrest dominated recurrent MI by a factor of 7 to 1. Dr. Haskell's review of the long-standing CAPRI program based in Seattle, Washington indicated that the complication rate was highest during the early years of the program, and that it decreased significantly in the later years. These changes probably reflected a combination of enhanced staff experience and expertise and improved patient selection.

PART 4

12

BIOCHEMICAL AND MUSCULAR
EFFECTS OF TRAINING

John O. Holloszy, M.D.

There is considerable information available regarding
the long-term adaptations that are induced in skeletal
muscle by endurance exercise such as long-distance running or swimming. The purpose of this article is to
review these adaptations and their possible physiological
role in the improvement in performance capacity that
frequently occurs in patients with ischemic heart disease
(ISCHD) in response to exercise training.

Adaptations Induced in Skeletal Muscle by Endurance Exercise

Most of the skeletal muscles in those mammalian species in which the adaptations to endurance exercise have
been studied are mixtures of three fiber types. These
are the fast-twitch white muscle fibers, which have a
low respiratory capacity, a high glycogenolytic capacity,
and high myosin ATPase activity; the fast-twitch red
fibers, which have a high respiratory capacity, a high
glycolytic capacity, and high myosin ATPase activity;
and the slow-twitch red fibers, which have a high respiratory capacity, a low glycogenolytic capacity, and
low myosin ATPase activity.[1] The red types of muscle,[2]
and particularly the slow-twitch red type of muscle in
humans,[3] are preferentially recruited during prolonged
exercise of moderate intensity requiring 65 to 80 percent
of VO_2 max. The magnitude of the adaptations induced in
muscle by endurance exercise is a function of contractile
activity.[4] In this context, it is not surprising that
the greatest adaptive responses to prolonged exercise of
moderate intensity are seen in the red muscle fibers.[1,5]

In addition to the biochemical adaptations, endurance exercise induces an increase in muscle capillaries which is reflected in an increase in the capillary per fiber ratio and in the number of capillaries around each fiber.[24,25]

Adaptive Response of Patients with Ischemic Heart Disease to Endurance Exercise

Healthy individuals who have a normal cardiovascular system undergo an adaptive increase in maximum cardiac output in response to endurance exercise training.[26-28] This adaptation contributes importantly to the increase in maximum O_2 uptake capacity (VO_2 max) induced by training.[26-28]

In contrast to normal individuals, studies on patients with ischemic heart disease have not shown any increase in maximal cardiac output in response to exercise training.[26,29-31] Nevertheless, many patients with ISCHD adapt to exercise with sizeable increases in VO_2 max and maximal work capacity.[28-33] This increase in VO_2 max in the absence of an increase in maximal cardiac output is achieved by an increased extraction of O_2 from the blood by the working muscles, as reflected in an increased arteriovenous O_2 difference.[28,29]

During submaximal exercise of the same intensity, oxygen uptake is usually unchanged, while cardiac output is lower, in patients with ISCHD after they have adapted to endurance exercise.[28,34,35] (The term "submaximal exercise" refers to work requiring less than VO_2 max.) In the trained patient with ISCHD, oxygen uptake is maintained, despite the lower cardiac output by increased O_2 extraction from the blood by the working muscles.[28-30,34] The physiological benefits of exercise training appear to be specific for exercise involving the muscle groups used in the training program; there appears to be little crossover adaptation of, for example, upper and lower extremity training effects.[28,32]

These findings provide evidence that in patients with ISCHD, both the increase in maximum exercise capacity and the increase in endurance during submaximal exercise are mediated by exercise-induced adaptations in the skeletal muscles and alterations in the responses of the endocrine and the autonomic systems to exercise[28,36] rather than by adaptations in the heart.

The most important biochemical adaptation of skeletal muscle to endurance exercise such as long distance running is an augmentation of respiratory capacity. This adaptation has been studied most extensively in rats; however, more recent muscle biopsy studies have confirmed that exercise training also induces increases in the respiratory capacity of skeletal muscle in man. Prolonged, intense training results in increases in the mitochondrial respiratory chain enzymes involved in the oxidation of NADH and succinate;[6,7,8,9] the enzymes of the citrate cycle;[10,11] mitochondrial ATPase (coupling factor 1), which catalyzes the oxidative phosphorylation of ADP to ATP;[12] the mitochondrial enzymes involved in the activation, transport, and beta-oxidation of fatty acids;[13] the enzymes involved in ketone oxidation;[5] and the enzymes of the malateasparate shuttle.[14] These increases in the levels of activity of a wide range of mitochondrial enzymes is due to an increase in enzyme protein. This is evidenced by an increase in the protein content of the mitochondrial fraction obtained from skeletal muscle and in the concentration of the cytochromes.[6,10]

Electron-microscopic studies on human and on rat skeletal muscles have provided evidence that both the size and number of muscle mitochondria increase in response to exercise.[8,15,16] Furthermore, exercise induces alterations in mitochondrial composition which tend to make skeletal muscle mitochondria more like heart mitochondria in their enzyme pattern.[1,5] In contrast to skeletal muscle, heart muscle, which is continually active, does not undergo an increase in respiratory capacity in response to endurance exercise.[17,18]

The increase in mitochondrial enzymes in skeletal muscle in response to exercise training is a rapid process. In rats subjected to a constant daily exercise stimulus, the increase in muscle mitochondria, as reflected in cytochrome c concentration and in the levels of activity of a number of mitochondrial enzymes, has a half-time of about 7 days.[19] The increase in the mitochondrial marker cytochrome c is preceded by an increase in beta-aminolevulinic acid synthetase activity.[20] Beta-aminolevulinic acid synthetase is the rate-limiting enzyme in heme synthesis, and it is our working hypothesis that the increase in this enzyme plays a key role in the increase in muscle mitochondria in response to exercise.[20]

Another biochemical adaptation to endurance exercise which may have important physiological consequences is an increase in muscle myoglobin concentration.[21,22] Myoglobin increases the rate of oxygen diffusion through a fluid layer,[23] and may facilitate oxygen utilization in muscle by increasing the rate of O_2 transport through the cytoplasm to the mitochondria.

References

1. Holloszy JO, Booth FW: Biochemical adaptations to endurance exercise in muscle. Ann Rev Physiol 38:273-291, 1976

2. Baldwin KM, Reitman JS, Terjung RL, Winder WW, Holloszy JO: Substrate depletion in different types of muscle and in liver during prolonged running. Am J Physiol 225:1045-1050, 1973

3. Gollnick PD, Armstrong RB, Saubert CW, Sembrowich WL, Shepherd RE, Saltin B: Glycogen depletion patterns in human skeletal muscle fibers during prolonged work. Pfluegers Arch 344:1-12, 1973

4. Fitts RH, Booth FW, Winder WW, Holloszy JO: Skeletal muscle respiratory capacity, endurance, and glycogen utilization. Am J Physiol 228:1029-1033, 1975

5. Winder WW, Baldwin KM, Holloszy JO: Enzymes involved in ketone utilization in different types of muscle: adaptation to exercise. Eur J Biochem 47:461-467, 1974

6. Holloszy JO: Biochemical adaptations in muscle. Effects of exercise on mitochondrial oxygen uptake and respiratory enzyme activity in skeletal muscle. J Biol Chem 242:2278-2282, 1967

7. Varnauskas E, Bjorntorp P, Fahlen M, Prerovsky I, Stenberg J: Effects of physical training on exercise blood flow and enzymatic activity in skeletal muscle. Cardiovasc Res 4:418-422, 1970

8. Morgan TE, Cobb LA, Short FA, Ross R, Gunn DR: Effect of long-term exercise on human muscle mitochondria. In, Muscle Metabolism During Exercise (Pernow B, Saltin B, eds). New York, Plenum, 1971, p 87

9. Bergman H, Bjorntorp P, Conradsson T-B, Fahlen M, Stenberg J, Varnauskas E: Enzymatic and circulatory adjustments to physical training in middle-aged men. Eur J Clin Lab Invest 3:414-418, 1973

10. Holloszy JO, Oscai LB, Don IJ, Mole PA: Mitochondrial citric acid cycle and related enzymes: adaptive response to exercise. Biochem Biophys Res Commun 40:1368-1373, 1970

11. Gollnick PD, Armstrong RB, Saltin B, Saubert CW IV, Sembrowich WL, Shepherd RE: Effect of training on enzyme activity and fiber composition of human skeletal muscle. J Appl Physiol 34:107-111, 1973

12. Oscai LB, Holloszy JO: Biochemical adaptations in muscle. II. Response of mitochondrial adenosine triphosphatase, creatine phosphokinase, and adenylate kinase activities in skeletal muscle to exercise. J Biol Chem 246:6968-6972, 1971

13. Mole PA, Oscai LB, Holloszy JO: Adaptation of muscle to exercise. Increase in levels of palmityl CoA synthetase, carnitine palmityltransferase, and palmityl CoA dehydrogenase and in the capacity to oxidize fatty acids. J Clin Invest 50:2323-2330, 1971

14. Holloszy JO: Adaptations of muscular tissue to training. Prog Cardiovasc Dis 18:445-458, 1976

15. Gollnick PD, King DW: Effect of exercise and training on mitochondria of rat skeletal muscle. Am J Physiol 216:1502-1509, 1969

16. Hoppeler H, Luthi P, Claassen H, Weibel ER, Howald H: The ultrastructure of normal human skeletal muscle. A morphometric analysis of untrained men, women and well-trained orienteers. Pfluegers Arch 344:217-232, 1973

17. Oscai LB, Mole PA, Brei B, Holloszy JO: Cardiac growth and respiratory enzyme levels in male rats subjected to a running program. Am J Physiol 220:1238-1241, 1971

18. Oscai LB, Mole PA, Holloszy JO: Effects of exercise on cardiac weight and mitochondria in male and female rats. Am J Physiol 220:1944-1948, 1971

19. Booth FW, Holloszy JO: Cytochrome c turnover in rat skeletal muscles. J Biol Chem 252:416-419, 1977

20. Holloszy JO, Winder WW: Induction of delta-aminolevulinic acid synthetase in muscle by exercise or thyroxine. Am J Physiol 236:R180-R183, 1979

21. Lawrie RA: Effect of enforced exercise on myoglobin concentration in muscle. Nature 171:1069-1970, 1953

22. Pattengale PK, Holloszy JO: Augmentation of skeletal muscle myoglobin by a program of treadmill running. Am J Physiol 213:783-785, 1967

23. Hemmingsen EA: Enhancement of oxygen transport by myoglobin. Comp Biochem Physiol 10:239-244, 1963

24. Brodal P, Ingjer F, Hermansen L: Capillary supply of skeletal muscle fibers in untrained and endurance-trained men. Am J Physiol 232:H705H712, 1977

25. Andersen P, Henricksson J: Capillary supply of the quadriceps muscle of man: adaptive response to exercise. J Physiol 270:677-690, 1977

26. Ekblom B, Astrand P-O, Saltin B, Stenberg J, Wallstrom B: Effect of training on circulatory response to exercise. J Appl Physiol 24:518, 1968

27. Rowell LB: Human cardiovascular adjustments to exercise and thermal stress. Physiol Rev 54:75-159, 1974

28. Clausen JP: Circulatory adjustments to dynamic exercise and effect of physical training in normal subjects and in patients with coronary artery disease. Prog Cardiovasc Dis 18, 459-495, 1976

29. Detry J-M, Rousseau M, Vandenbroucke G, Kusumi F, Brasseur LA, Bruce RA: Increased arteriovenous oxygen difference after physical training in coronary heart disease. Circulation 44:109-118, 1971

30. Rousseau MF, Brasseur LA, Detry J-M: Hemodynamic determinants of maximal oxygen intake in patients with healed myocardial infarction; influence of physical training. Circulation 48:943-949, 1973

31. Clausen JP, Trap-Jensen J: In, Coronary Heart Disease and Physical Fitness (Larsen OA, Malmborg RO, eds). Copenhagen, Munksgaard, 1971, p 74

32. Hellerstein HK: Limitations of marathon running in the rehabilitation of coronary patients: anatomic and physiological determinants. Ann NY Acad Sci 301:484-494, 1977

33. Kavanagh T, Shephard RJ, Kennedy J: Characteristics of post-coronary marathon runners. Ann NY Acad Sci 301:455-465, 1977

34. Varnauskas E, Bergman H, Houk P, Bjorntorp P: Haemodynamic effects of physical training in coronary patients. Lancet 2:8-12, 1966

35. Clausen JP, Larsen OA, Trap-Jensen J: Physical training in the management of coronary artery disease. Circulation 40:143-154, 1969

36. Hartley LH, Mason JW, Hogan RP, Jones LG, Kotchen TA, Mougey EH, Wherry FE, Pennington LL, Ricketts PT: Multiple hormonal responses to prolonged exercise in relation to physical training. J Appl Physiol 33:607-610, 1972

13

PHYSICAL TRAINING IN PATIENTS WITH INTERMITTENT CLAUDICATION

Bengt Saltin, M.D.

Introduction

As early as 1898, Erb[1] suggested increased physical activity in the form of walking as treatment for intermittent claudication (CI). This recommendation had not been followed to any great extent until the last 2 decades, but now, especially in Scandinavia, it is a common practice to recommend that patients with milder forms of CI "train." Numerous studies are now available evaluating the clinical results as well as the underlying mechanisms for the improved walking tolerance so frequently observed as the result of active participation in a training regimen.

In this article, a short summary of these different studies will be given as well as some comments about the feasibility of training patients with intermittent claudication. The main focus, however, will be on the physiological and biochemical changes of the leg skeletal muscle observed in CI patients as a result of training.

Walking Tolerance

Larsen and Lassen[2] were among the first to demonstrate a significant improvement in walking tolerance in patients with intermittent claudication. Similar findings have been obtained in a great number of studies.[3-19] It is customary to observe a doubling in walking distance after 2 to 3 months of training with 2 to 3 weekly sessions of 30 to 60 min duration.

Of note is that the patients chosen for physical training are carefully selected. For example, severe cases with ulcer or with such a low level of leg blood flow that there is an obvious risk for an ulceration are not considered for this type of treatment. The same is usually true for patients with pain in the leg at rest. Thus, patients in whom the ischemic pain appears after some minutes of walking but is severe enough to call for a pause are advised to enhance their physical activity. Studies reported upon in this article have used either plethysmographic measurements of postischemic calf blood flow or blood pressure drop between arm and ankle or toe to verify that the poor walking capacity is due to a low blood flow to the lower extremities.

The occlusion can be high (aorta or a. ilica) or low (a. femoralis) in the arterial tree, and it has been thought that patients with low occlusions respond best to physical training. This notion may not be right. Ekroth and coworkers[20] have found in their large body of material that in patients with low and high occlusions, there is a significant improvement in walking distance, which is of the same relative magnitude in both groups.

Similar results were noted by Jonason et al.[12] Thirteen patients with proximal stenosis almost doubled walking tolerance after the 3 months (from 347 m to 687 m) and 23 patients with distal stenosis improved their maximal walking tolerance from 440 m to 666 m. Comparisons have been made between supervised (hospital) and self-administered (home) training. The supervised training gave the best results.[6,14] However, there are several reasons why a continuous training regimen has to be self-administered. Positive results are also available with 1 to 3 months' organized training followed by self-administered training when the patients first are accustomed to the need for physical activity and know how it should be executed.

Results are available from a study in which the supervised introduction period was 1 (12 x 1 hr) or 3 months (30 x 1 hr), after which the CI patients administered their training themselves.[8] The maximal walking tolerance improved only a little with 1 month of training, but a gradual, continuous further improvement was noticed also in the patient group, who self-administered their training. Thus, after 6 months, both groups were approximately 14 percent better, i.e., maximal walking distance was increased from approximately 170 (160 to 177) m to 430 (426 to 431) m. After 1 year, a declining trend was observed, but in both groups, walking tolerance was still twice the length it was before the training started.[8]

One study[12] has included CI patients with pain at rest or angina pectoris. In the former group, which consisted of eight patients, rather positive results were observed after 3 months of training. Six of them improved walking distance considerably, and their rest pain diminished or disappeared. The other two patients' performance was unchanged. Of the 24 CI patients who also had coronary insufficiency, 14 improved their walking distance from 450 m to 736 m. The remaining 10 patients worsened and maximal walking distance dropped by 100 m to 406 m. Also, CI patients with gangrene have successfully gone through a training regimen.[21]

The training programs contain a predominance of leg exercises to improve flexibility, strength, and endurance of the leg muscles, especially the calf muscles. After warming-up periods, various forms of walking are performed; for example, folk dancing has proved to be stimulating and successful. Any special emphasis on intensity in the training is seldom of importance, whereas encouragement to continue the training is needed, especially for those who train at home. Regular followup tests of walking tolerance can stimulate patients to a better adherence, and medical reasons may also speak in favor of retesting at 6- or 12-month intervals.

Mechanisms for Improved Walking Tolerance

There are three basic mechanisms by which walking tolerance can be improved. They are: better technique for walking, thereby reducing the energy demand at a given walking speed (mechanical efficiency); enhanced anaerobic energy yield, possibly combined with increased tolerance to withstand ischemic pain; and increased oxygen supply.

Mechanical efficiency

Two different approaches have been used to elucidate whether walking and other forms of enhanced physical activity affect the technique of walking. Carlsoo and coworkers[22] demonstrated that the vertical and the sagittal and transverse horizontal forces on a force platform did not differ much when CI patients were compared to controls. Further, no changes were observed in the patient group with training. Oxygen uptake and blood lactate concentration at walking speeds no higher than 4 km/hr could be tolerated by the patients for 8 to 10 min both before and after a training period, indicating no significant drop in oxygen uptake. Blood lactate concentration was slightly lower after the training, but the magnitude of change is barely of significance for the total energy turnover and thus for the mechanical efficiency. These studies, then, indicate that a change in the gait and in oxygen demand is not an important factor in explaining an improved walking tolerance after training.

In contrast to these findings stand the clinical observations that CI patients walk better after the training. It has been suggested that an elevation of the step frequency plays a role.[15] The possibility may exist that quicker contractions may not affect the biomechanics of the gait or the energy demand very much, but that the limited blood flow is better utilized.[15]

Anaerobic capacity and ischemic pain tolerance

<u>Anaerobic energy yield</u>. The more restricted the blood flow is to the leg, the more important will be the anaerobic energy yield in the skeletal muscle for work performance. Lactate is also produced and accumulates at low exercise intensities in patients with CI, and with ischemic pain, large quantities of anaerobic metabolites are found in the muscle. In light of these facts, it is surprising that CI patients do not have a high anaerobic capacity and that an enhancement of this capacity is not observed with training. CI patients cannot perform ischemic work (tourniquet around arm or leg) better than controls. In addition, muscle and blood lactate concentrations are not especially high in exhaustive exercise performed by CI patients compared with controls. Muscle ATP depletion is also normal, whereas the CP depletion may be slightly more pronounced than in controls at exhaustion.[23] After a period of training, no changes in these variables are observed.[24]

Another sign of unchanged skeletal muscle anaerobic potential after training is that the activity of glycolytic enzymes is similar in CI patients and controls both before[25,26] and after a period of training.[26] It thus appears that the maximum amount of energy liberated by anaerobic means is the same after as before training and that an enhanced anaerobic energy yield does not contribute to an increased walking distance.

Is there an explanation why CI patients are not distinguished by a high anaerobic capacity? There is no obvious answer. Several factors influence the energy yield from anaerobic processes (only the lactacid component is considered, as any difference in depletion of the phosphagen stores must be of very minor importance from a quantitative standpoint). The three main factors to be considered are rate of production of lactate, its elimination, and the capacity to accumulate lactate of H^+ in the muscle cell. The absolute rate of the glycolysis is most likely not extremely high at exhaustive

exercise in CI patients, as the contractions performed
are not very forceful, nor are they repeated with a high
frequency.

The ADP/ATP ratio appears to be the same as in controls.[23] Of the formed pyruvate, some is oxidized and
some is reduced to lactate. Due to the limited availability of oxygen, a substantial fraction of the pyruvate
is converted to lactate. For the same reason only very
little of this lactate can be converted to pyruvate and
oxidized in adjacent muscle cells (slow twitch oxidative
fibers). The release of lactate from the muscle is flow-
dependent. The perfusion of the leg skeletal muscle in
CI patients is low[23,27] and so is the lactate elimination.[23] The capacity to buffer the metabolic acidosis in
the muscle or blood is probably the same in CI patients
and controls.

Of the above-described events, training may effect the
perfusion, which may mean that during the exhaustive exercise, more pyruvate is oxidized and more lactate can
be released from the exercising muscles. As discussed
below, the increase in muscle blood flow is small and in
many patients nonexistent.

Endurance training in healthy man does not influence
the level of the glycolytic enzymes, while extreme sprint
training does.[28] It may be, then, that the rate of glycolysis is too slow in CI patients in training to be a
stimulus for an enhancement of the enzymes in glycolytic
pathways.

Ischemic pain. Could it be that instead of markedly
improving the anaerobic capacity, training prepares the
CI patient to better tolerate the metabolic changes in
the leg muscles during a tolerance test? One indication
that this is not the case is the finding of similar subjective ratings of discomfort during a tolerance test
of CI patients before and after training.[10] The onset
of pain and the point at which it becomes intolerable
were experienced at equal levels of improvement, i.e.,
after training, the walking distance to onset of pain and
to intolerable pain are prolonged by the same amount,
300 to 400 m.

There is further proof that ischemic pain tolerance
is not changed. Onset of pain and point of exhaustion
occurred before and after training at similar muscle
lactate, ATP, and CP concentrations, but the work performed (equal work time) was much greater. That means
that the rate of depletion of the phosphagens and the
accumulation of lactate during the exercise were slower.
However, when the changes in these compounds reached a
certain level, which was the same before and after training, onset of pain and exhaustion occurred. Possibly

none of the compounds (lactate, ATP, or CP) have a causal relationship with the sensation of pain. However, they appear to be closely associated with the subjective feeling of fatigue and pain.[29,30]

In this context, it must be pointed out that the cause of ischemic pain is unknown. High muscle lactate (and pH and osmolality), ADP, and P_i concentration can probably be ruled out, along with low ATP and CP levels, as they do not differ at the end of short-term exhaustive exercise in controls and in CI patients. The latter group experienced the typical ischemic pain. Other causes for ischemic pain, although not investigated, are AMP and K^+. The AMP concentration in the cell should be related to the ADP concentration and can then be expected to be neither very high nor different in controls and CI patients.[31] What is left, then, is K^+, which might be the most likely candidate. Intense muscular contractions result in a flux of K^+ out of the muscle cell.[22] With a low leg blood flow, a large amount of the K^+ will accumulate in the interstitial space.[32,33] The receptors, in the form of free nerve endings, are also located here.

Results of bicycle exercise in patients with CI should be looked upon with the same caution. For one thing, the work performed in a pedal thrust by the calf muscles as compared to the thigh muscles to a large extent depends upon where the foot is placed on the pedal. Only if the front of the foot is placed on the pedal will the calf muscles markedly contribute to work performance.[34]

Another important factor is that in pedalling the bicycle, the force developed can be unevenly distributed between the legs. If the work tests are performed on a bicycle, the feet must be properly placed on the pedals using no clips, and the strain gauges must be mounted to the pedals so that one can ascertain an equal application of force during each pedal thrust.

Leg muscle O_2 supply

An improvement in the O_2 supply to the leg can occur either by widening the $A-VO_2$ difference or by increasing the blood flow or by a combination of both factors.

Muscle blood flow. Plethysmographic measurements can only be applied at rest, and results from postischemic flow measurements may not directly apply to the situation during normal walking. The Xe^{132} method can be applied during exercise, but its value as a quantitative measure of muscle blood flow is questionable. These methodological problems contribute to the uncertainty about possible changes in muscle blood flow after training in CI patients. There are studies showing an increase in flow, whereas others have shown no increase.[2-4,7,16,35,36]

186

In the well-controlled studies of CI patients by Schersten and coworkers,[5,35] muscle blood flow was elevated in some patients, whereas other patients revealed no increase in flow. An improved perfusion appeared not to be essential for increasing the walking distance, as there was a substantial increase in all patients. This finding has recently been confirmed using the thermodilution technique to measure lower leg blood flow.[17] Walking distance was unchanged or increased in the ten patients, the mean increase being 78 percent, whereas the flow did not change (-8 percent; range -31 to 17 percent).

If a reduced blood pressure difference between arm and toe is taken as an indicator of a better perfusion, the picture is still the same. Small or no changes in the pressure difference have been observed with training, but improvement in walking distance has always been shown.[14]

Soon after an occlusion of an artery to the leg, there may be a development of collaterals.[37-39] Thus the possibility exists that if the training regimen starts close enough to the appearance of a stenosis, an increased flow to the leg will be registered, whereas training in a later phase of CI is less likely to affect the collateral development. To what extent variation in the time of the start of training is related to the onset of the disease is not known. It may be that the influence of training on the leg muscle blood flow is on a more favorable distribution of the flow rather than affecting the arterial inflow.

Leg $A-VO_2$ difference. Zetterqvist[40] has shown that the leg $A-VO_2$ difference is high during intense exercise in CI patients but that a further extraction of oxygen occurs as the result of a training regimen. Unfortunately, the practical importance of this widening of the $A-VO_2$ difference is flow-dependent, i.e., with a low blood flow, little is gained in absolute terms, and with a high flow, large quantities of oxygen are made available for the cell. At exhaustive exercise in a healthy middle-aged man, leg blood flow (one leg) may be 6 l/min[41] as compared to 0.5 to 1.5 l/min in a CI patient.[23,27]

Physical training may enhance leg blood flow from 0.25 to 0.50 l/min in CI patients at the very most, while the $A-VO_2$ difference is widened with 2 vol/percent.[17,41] In leg oxygen uptake, these increases represent only 0.02 l/min for the two legs. Although these estimates are based on leg blood flow determinations, which may represent only 1/3 to 2/3 of the total flow to the leg,[17,41] it is apparent that the absolute increase in the volume of oxygen made available to and used by the legs is quite small.

In recent years, methods have been made available for morphological and biochemical studies of small muscle tissue samples obtained by a needle. Some of these methods have also been used with CI patients in connection with training.

Capillaries. In CI patients, the number of capillaries expressed per mm^2 or per fiber is the same or slightly higher than those found in age-matched controls.[42] The mean area of the fibers is normal, which means that the calculated average area each capillary has to supply is the same or slightly smaller than in the controls.[42] The changes in capillarization observed after a couple of months of training are small, but the trends are clear.[43]

The fiber area is slightly larger but the number of capillaries around each fiber has increased to such an extent that the calculated average area for each capillary to supply is smaller. This rather rich supply of capillaries may explain the large A-VO$_2$ difference found in CI patients when exercising. With a dense capillary network, the capillary blood volume is high. With a low muscle blood flow, mean transit time for the red cells in the capillaries will be quite long, allowing for a more complete diffusion of the oxygen to the cells.

The above discussion is based on a normal function of the capillaries in leg muscles of CI patients. Whether this is the case can be questioned. The histochemical visualization of the capillaries has revealed that, especially in severe cases of claudication, many capillaries have an abnormal appearance.[43] The basal membrane of these capillaries is markedly thickened.[44,45]

In addition, some of the capillaries may be closed.[46] Based on these observations, it may be that the degree of capillarization in the leg muscle of CI patients may not be that favorable. A period of training bringing about a capillary proliferation can then be critical and aid in redistributing the minimal flow available and reducing the diffusion distance to the muscle fibers most active in the exercise.

Oxidative enzymes. Schersten and colleagues have reported a high activity for various mitochondrial enzymes in the leg skeletal muscle of CI patients.[9,47-51] According to these authors, the functional significance of this adaptation to the disease is that it brings about the widening of the leg A-VO$_2$ difference. As previously discussed, the capillarization of the muscle probably plays a greater role for the observed large oxygen extraction than changes in mitochondrial volume and oxidative enzymes of the muscles. Moreover, it is questionable whether CI patients have higher oxidative enzyme levels than age-matched healthy controls.[42]

In the study of Schersten et al.,[9,47-51] the control subjects were patients in a surgical ward. When a control group of healthy untrained subjects is chosen, lower rather than higher activity for oxidative enzymes is found in the CI patients. The best proof that a reduced blood flow to a leg does not enhance the activities of the oxidative enzymes is the finding in the rare CI patients with an occlusion in only one leg[42] that the succinate dehydrogenase and cytochrome-c-oxidase activities are the same in the occluded as in the unoccluded leg. In addition, this activity level was slightly lower in the CI patients than in the healthy, untrained age-matched controls.

There are also other studies demonstrating subnormal oxidative potentials in the leg muscles of CI patients.[18,26] As an argument against this opinion, results from morphometric analysis of the mitochondrial volume in muscle fibers of CI patients have been used. These studies revealed slightly larger mitochondrial volume in muscle fibers of m. tibialis anterior in the most affected or symptomatic leg.[54] The quantification of mitochondrial volume was performed only on muscle fibers with no signs of degeneration.

The number of pathological fibers was highest in the most symptomatic leg. Thus, large mitochondrial volume and low oxidative capacity may not be incompatible findings. In the most symptomatic leg, the oxidative capacity of the normal muscle fibers is "diluted" by the degenerated fibers, and the measurement of the activity of mitochondrial enzymes on the whole-muscle homogenate will come out low. In addition to this explanation, the possibility always exists that the oxidative enzyme content is not directly related to the mitochondrial volume.

There is a coupling between the activity of the enzymes in a metabolic pathway and the capacity for a substrate flux through that pathway.[52] With training of CI patients, leg skeletal muscle glycolytic enzymes are unchanged and low,[24] while enzymes in the beta-oxidation and tricarboxylic acid cycles as well as the respiratory chain are enhanced.[9,18,27,49] In CI patients before training, the use of FFA during exercise is low and the anaerobic metabolism considerable.[53]

After training, a larger use of FFA can be expected and more of the formed pyruvate can be oxidized; both changes reduce the need for lactate formation. That less lactate is produced at a given exercise intensity after training in CI patients is a common finding. In vitro studies of incorporation of glucose in various metabolites can be taken as an indicator of altered pattern of metabolic activity.[5,42,48,49]

The finding of a larger glucose-carbon incorporation in CO_2 after training indicates a greater contribution of the mitochondria to the ATP resynthesis.[48] In vivo studies are needed, however, to elucidate the more exact role of the changed metabolic potential of the leg skeletal muscle of CI patients after training. This is especially true in order to be able to quantify the functional significance of the metabolic adaptation for improved walking tolerance.

For an enhancement of the rate of oxidation, the oxygen supply must be elevated. As a larger $A-VO_2$ difference can play only a very minor role during intense exercise in CI patients, there must be an increase in the blood flow to the muscle fibers where the rate of oxidation is increased. The importance of the small changes in the pattern for the metabolic potentials observed after training in CI patients may be negligible in comparison to a slightly better blood supply. Of note also is that with a better perfusion of the muscle fibers with the highest metabolic rate, more lactate can be released from the muscle.

Concluding Remarks

Patients with mild forms of CI do benefit from participating in a training regimen. A walking distance which may be only 100-200 m before training can be elevated to 400 m or more after training. The increase in walking distance before any pain is felt is of at least the same magnitude as the improvement in maximal walking distance.

These improvements mean that the CI patients can perform daily routine activities with less discomfort. Two to 3 hours of physical activity per week appear to be needed to give substantial improvements within a couple of months. This "training" should, at least in the beginning, be supervised. To obtain a high adherence to the training regimen when it is self-administered, regular followup may be beneficial.

In fact, only minimal or no changes may have been observed in any of the three factors--mechanical efficiency, anaerobic, and aerobic energy yields--which can cause work performance to become elevated. This is an apparent paradox that may be explicable in part.

Work performance is determined on the basis of time or distance at a preset speed and inclination on the treadmill. A CI patient walks before training a 4 km/hr and 5° inclination to exhaustion. His oxygen uptake is 1.2 l/min as compared to a demand of 1.9 l/min with his present walking technique. With an anaerobic capacity equivalent to 2.8 l/min O_2, he can tolerate the exercise for not more than 3.5 to 4 min.

After the training, the energy demand at the same speed and inclination is 1.8 l/min (mechanical efficiency improved 5.2 percent). His oxygen uptake has increased 0.14 l/min (14 percent combined effect of increased blood flow and widened A-VO_2 difference) to 1.34 l/min, and the total amount of energy that can be liberated by anaerobic means is elevated to the equivalent of 3.2 l/min of oxygen (14 percent combined effect of improved anaerobic capacity and higher ischemic pain threshold).

In this latter case, work time will be around 7 min. In other words, small changes in each of the factors of importance for work performance are sufficient to explain a doubling of the maximal walking distance. In the individual case, the possibility also exists that only one or two of the discussed mechanisms are changed, but the order of magnitude of the changes must then be greater. Thus, in order to account for the better work performance in CI patients after training, a multifactorial approach is needed. Presently, results from such studies are not available. When they are, the apparent paradox mentioned earlier may no longer exist.

Acknowledgements

The work on this subject,[8,24,26,42,43] which has been performed at the A. Krogh Institute, was made possible by financial support from the Danish Heart Association and the Wahral Science Research Council.

References

1. Erb W: Uber das "intermitterende Hinken" und nervose Storungen in Folge vom Gefasserkrankungen. Dtsch Z Nervenheilkunde 13:1, 1898

2. Larsen OA, Lassen NA: Effect of daily muscular exercise in patients with intermittent claudication. Lancet II:1093, 1966

3. Alpert JS, Larsen JS, Lassen NA: Exercise and intermittent claudication. Blood flow in the calf muscle during walking studied by the Xenon-133 clearance method. Circulation 39:353, 1969

4. Cachovan M, Maries HD, Kunitsch G: Einfluss von Intervalltraining auf die Leistungsfahigkeit und periphere Durchblutung bei Patienten mit Claudicatio Intermittens. Z Kardiol 65:54, 1976

5. Dahllof A-G: Perifer arteriel insufficiens i nedre extremiteterne. Goteborg, Avhandling, 1975

6. Egelund B, Wenkens, Nielsen SL, Prahl M: A comparison of supervised and self-administered training in patients with claudicatio intermittens. (In Danish) Dansk fysiot 20:11, 1976

7. Ericsson B, Haeger K, Lindell S-E: Effect of physical training on intermittent claudication. Angiology 21:188, 1970

8. Grunnert J, Roldsgaard T: Training ability and interest in physical training in patients with claudicatio intermittens. (In Danish). Master's thesis 128, A Krogh Inst, Copenhagen Univ, 1979

9. Holm J, Dahllof A-G, Bjorntorp P, Schersten T: Enzyme studies in muscles of patients with intermittent claudication. Effect of training. Scand J Clin Lab Invest 31:201, 1973

10. Holm J, Schersten T: Metabolic change in skeletal muscles after physical conditioning and in peripheral arterial insufficiency. Swed J Def Med 10:71, 1974

11. Hovind H, Basboll Holm A, Holstein P, Levin Nielsen S: Daily walking in intermittent claudication. (In Danish) Ugeskr Laeg 138:90, 1976

12. Jonason T, Jonzon B, Ringqvist I, Oman-Rydberg A: Effect of physical training on different categories of patients with intermittent claudication. Acta Med Scand 206:253, 1979

13. McAllister FF: The fate of patients with intermittent claudication managed nonoperatively. Am J Surg 132:593, 1976

14. Nielsen SL, Larsen B, Prahl M, Jensen CT: Hospitals-traening contra hjemmetraening af patienter med claudicatio intermittens. Ugeskr Laeg Nr 46: 2733, 1977

15. Schoop W: Mechanism of beneficial action of daily walking training of patients with intermittent claudication. Scand J Clin Lab Invest, suppl 128, 31:197, 1973

16. Skinner JS, Strandness JDE: Exercise and intermittent claudication. II. Effect of physical training. Circulation 36:23, 1967

17. Sorlie D, Myhre K: Effects of physical training in intermittent claudication. Scand J Clin Invest 38: 217, 1978

18. Valtola J, Hanninen O: Muscular metabolism in chronic cardiovascular disease and effects of programmed training. Pubs Univ of Kuopio (Finland) 1:7, 1976

19. Zetterqvist S: The effect of active training on nutritive blood flow in exercising ischemic legs. Scand J Clin Lab Invest 24:101, 1970

20. Ekroth R, Dahllof A-G, Gundevall B, Holm J, Schersten T: Physical training of patients with intermittent claudication: indications, methods, and results. Surgery 84:640, 1978

21. Foley WT: Treatment of gangrene of the feet and legs by walking. Circulation XV:689, 1957

22. Carlsoo S, Dahllof A-G, Holm J: Kinetic analysis of the gait in patients with hemiparesis and in patients with intermittent claudication. Scand J Rehab Med 6:166, 1974

23. Pernow B, Saltin B, Wahren J, Cronestrand R, Ekestrom S: Leg blood flow and muscle metabolism in occlusive arterial disease of the leg before and after reconstructive surgery. Clin Sci Mol Med 49:265, 1975

24. Molander B, Mygind E: Metabolic changes in m. gastrocnemius of CI patients with exercise, with a note on the effect of training. Master's thesis 114, A Krogh Inst, Copenhagen Univ, 1978

25. Falholt K, Dohn K, Lund B, Falholt W: Enzyme pattern in hypoxic skeletal muscle. J Mol Cell Cardiol 6:349, 1974

26. Skjellerup N, Gutheil F: Capillary density and enzyme activities in m. gastrocnemius in CI patients, with a note on the effect of physical training. Master's thesis 111, A Krogh Inst, Copenhagen Univ, 1978

27. Sorlie D, Myhre K: Lower leg blood flow in inter-
    mittent claudication. Scand J Clin Invest 38:171,
    1978

28. Saltin B, Henriksson J, Nygaard E, Andersen P,
    Jansson E: Fiber types and metabolic potentials of
    skeletal muscles in sedentary man and endurance
    runners. Ann NY Acad Sci 391:3, 1977

29. Borg G: Simple rating methods for estimation of
    perceived exertion. Physical work and effort.
    Oxford, Pergamon Press, 1977

30. Karlsson J, Saltin B: Lactate, ATP, and CP in work-
    ing muscles during exhaustive exercise in man. J
    Appl Physiol 29:598, 1970

31. McGilvery RW: The use of fuels for muscular work.
    In, Metabolic Adaptation to Prolonged Physical
    Exercise (Howald H, Poortmans JR, eds). Basel,
    Birkhauser Verlag, 1973, p 12

32. Hnik P, Holas M, Krekule J, Kriz N, Mejsnar A,
    Smiesko V, Kjec E, Vyskocil F: Work-induced potas-
    sium changes in skeletal muscle and effluent venous
    blood assessed by liquid ion-exchanger micro-elec-
    trodes. Pfluegers Arch 362:85, 1976

33. Sjogaard G, Saltin B: Changes in intra- and extra-
    cellular muscle water contents and electrolyte
    concentrations in man during intense exercise.
    Acta Physiol Scand (suppl) 473:80

34. Petersen FB: Physical performance capacity and lo-
    cal haemodynamics in dysbasia arteriosclerotica.
    Copenhagen, Danmark Theois, 1974

35. Dahllof A-G, Holm J, Schersten T, Sivertsson R:
    Peripheral arterial insufficiency, effect of physi-
    cal training on walking tolerance, calf blood flow
    and blood flow resistance. Scand J Rehab Med 8:19,
    1976

36. Lassen NA, Larsen OA: Effect of training on the
    circulation in ischemic muscle tissue. Observations
    of calf muscle blood flow in patients with intermit-
    tent claudication and a discussion of the myocardial
    blood flow changes in patients with angina pectoris.
    In, Coronary Heart Disease and Physical Fitness
    (Larsen OA, Malmborg R, eds). Copenhagen,
    Munksgaard, 1971, p 163

37. Broome A, Cederlund J, Eklof B: Spontaneous re-
    covery in intermittent claudication. Scand J Clin
    Lab Invest (suppl) 99:157, 1967

38. Eckstein RW: Effect of exercise and coronary artery narrowing on collateral circulation. Circ Res 5: 230, 1957

39. Sanne H, Sivertsson R: The effect of exercise on the development of collateral circulation after experimental occlusion of the femoral artery in the calf. Acta Physiol Scand 73:257, 1968

40. Zetterqvist S: Effect of training in intermittent claudication. Redistribution of blood flow due to training. In, Coronary Heart Disease and Physical Fitness (Larson OA, Malmborg RO, eds). Munksgaard, Copenhagen, 1971, pp 158-162

41. Wahren J, Jorfeldt L: Determination of leg blood flow during exercise in man: an indicator dilution technique based on femoral venous dye infusion. Clin Sci Mol Med 45:135, 1973

42. Henriksson J, Nygaard E, Andersson J, Eklof B: Peripheral arterial insufficiency: fibre types, capillarization and enzyme activities in patients with intermittent claudication. Scand J Clin Lab Invest 10, 1980

43. Nygaard E, Gutheil F, Henriksson J, Saltin B: Capillary density and oxidative periarteritis in the gastrocnemius muscle of patients with claudication. Scand J Clin Lab Invest, 1980 (in press)

44. Makitie J: Skeletal muscle capillaries in intermittent claudication. Arch Pathol Lab Med 101:500, 1977

45. Makitie J, Teravainen H: Muscle microvasculature in arteriosclerosis obliterans. Acta Neuro Pathol, 1980 (in press)

46. Fagrell B: Vital capillaroscopy. A clinical method for studying changes of skin microcirculation in patients suffering from vascular disorders of the leg. Angiology 23:284, 1972

47. Bylund AC, Hammarsten J, Holm J, Schersten T: Enzyme activities in skeletal muscles from patients with peripheral arterial insufficiency. Eur J Clin Invest 6:425, 1976

48. Dahllof A-G, Bjorntorp P, Holm J, Schersten T: Metabolic activity of skeletal muscle in patients with peripheral arterial insufficiency. Eur J Invest 4:9, 1974

49. Holm J: Skeletal muscle metabolism in patients with peripheral arterial insufficiency. Thesis. Goteborg, Sweden, 1972

50. Holm J, Bjorntorp P, Schersten T: Metabolic activity in human skeletal muscle. Effect of peripheral arterial insufficiency. Eur J Clin Invest 2:321, 1972

51. Holm J, Dahllof A-G, Schersten T: Metabolic activity of skeletal muscle in patients with peripheral arterial insufficiency. Scand J Clin Lab Invest 35:81-86, 1975

52. Holloszy J-O, Booth FW: Biochemical adaptations to endurance exercise in muscle. Ann Rev Physiol 38: 273, 1976

53. Hagenfeldt L, Wahren J, Pernow B, Cronestrand R, Ekestrom S: Free fatty acid metabolism of leg muscles during exercise in patients with obliterative iliac and femoral artery disease before and after reconstructive surgery. J Clin Invest 51: 3061, 1972

54. Angquist K-A: Human skeletal muscle fibre structure. Effects of physical training and arterial insufficiency. Umea Univ Med Dissertations, New Series No 39, Umea, 1978

14

HEMODYNAMIC AND METABOLIC EFFECTS OF BETA-ADRENOCEPTOR BLOCKADE ON SKELETAL MUSCLE DURING EXERCISE

Anders C. Juhlin-Dannfelt, M.D.

Beta-adrenoceptor blockade induces a variety of cardio-vascular and metabolic changes. The central hemodynamic effects--such as a reduced heart rate, cardiac output, and blood pressure--are well known. The beta-adrenergic system is also involved in local vascular changes and substrate supply to the muscles. Thus, beta-blockade could induce important changes in muscle metabolism, especially during exercise.

In healthy men, maximal oxygen uptake is unchanged or only slightly reduced by beta-blockade, despite a decrease in heart rate of 30-40 beats/min. However, the time for a maximal run or bicycle work is reduced by as much as 25 percent.[1,2] There are also data available indicating that the capacity to perform prolonged submaximal exercise is reduced.[3,4] Furthermore, a well-known side effect of beta-blockade treatment is muscular fatigue. Since an increasing number of patients are being treated with long-term beta-blockade, it seems of importance to take into consideration the peripheral muscular effects. This review will deal with some recent data on how adrenoceptor blockade influences muscle blood flow, oxygen uptake, and substrate utilization during exercise and on the effect of training.

Leg Blood Flow and Oxygen Uptake

During exercise, there is a linear relationship between leg blood flow and workload, i.e., at a given load, the flow is within narrow limits in healthy subjects.[5] During treatment with propranolol, leg blood flow is decreased both in hypertensives[6] and in healthy subjects (Juhlin-Dannfelt et al., to be published). The decrease in leg blood flow is about the same in magnitude as the decrease in cardiac output, i.e., the relationship of leg blood flow/cardiac output is unchanged. One question in this context is whether the peripheral vascular B_2-receptors in the skeletal muscles are of any importance for regulating blood flow during exercise. A way to study this is to induce a local beta-blockade in one leg. This can be achieved by giving the drug slowly in the femoral artery.[7] By using a low dose of propranolol (2 mg), systemic effects are avoided and heart rate is unchanged. Evidence for a local blockade in the leg is that when epinephrine is given intravenously at a rate of 0.1 g/kg/min, no increase in leg blood flow is seen in the blocked leg, whereas in the leg with unblocked beta-receptors, the flow is more than doubled, with a decrease in the vascular resistance. During exercise, however, the flow is exactly the same whether or not the beta-receptors are blocked. These results clearly indicate that local factors other than the B_2-receptors are responsible for the exercise-induced vasodilation.

The lower blood flow to the working muscles during systemic beta-blockade means a reduced capacity to transport oxygen. However, earlier studies have shown that at a given workload, pulmonary oxygen uptake is not significantly changed by blockade.[1,2,6] This favors the possibility of an unchanged uptake of oxygen by the muscles. Support for this possibility is provided by the finding that during submaximal exercise, between 30-90 percent of max VO_2, the extraction of oxygen from the femoral vein is increased sufficiently to compensate for the lower blood flow, resulting in an unchanged or only slightly reduced oxygen uptake (Juhlin-Dannfelt et al., to be published). Thus, it appears that at submaximal exercise, a reduced oxygen supply is not the explanation for an impaired endurance.

Substrate Use

The adrenergic system is important for the regulation of two of the major substrates for the muscles, namely the free fatty acids (FFA) and glycogen. Beta-adrenergic receptor blockade in therapeutic doses inhibits lipolysis, resulting in a reduction of blood FFA to about 50-70 percent of normal.[8,9] Since lipolysis is mediated by the B_1-receptors, both selective and unselective blocking drugs reduce blood FFA concentration.[10]

In man, the uptake of FFA by the exercising limb muscles rises in direct proportion to the arterial inflow, expressed as the product of arterial concentration and

plasma flow.[11] Since, during beta-blockade, both flow
and concentration of FFA are reduced, less substrate is
available, and the working muscles must depend on carbohydrate as an energy source.

Glycogenolysis in the muscles can be facilitated by
catecholamines or by contraction, with both activating
phosphorylase a. The mechanism of activation of phosphorylase by muscle contraction is basically different
from that involving adrenergic amines.[12,13] With beta-
adrenoceptor blockade, the epinephrine-induced glycogenolysis can be totally inhibited. The role of the catecholamines in muscle glycogen depletion during exercise
is not clear, and studies have shown both decreased[14,15]
and increased[3] rates of glycogen breakdown when the beta-
adrenergic receptors are blocked. To further elucidate
the effect of beta-blockade on glycogen breakdown during
exercise, we gave propranolol intraperitoneally to rats
in a dose of 1 mg/kg body weight. This is a dose sufficient to completely block catecholamine-induced glycogen
breakdown, even when a high dose of epinephrine is given
subcutaneously (1 mg/kg body weight). Figure 1 shows
the glycogen content in the different rat muscles in

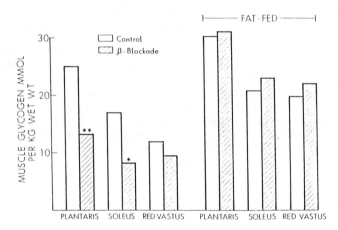

Figure 1. Muscle glycogen concentrations after 1 hour
of exercise in rats given propranolol ▨ or saline ▢
intraperitoneally. The right half of the figure shows
glycogen concentration in the fat-fed animals.

blocked and unblocked animals after 55 minutes of strenuous exercise on a treadmill. The data clearly show
that glycogen breakdown during exercise is not inhibited
by beta-adrenoceptor blockade. Instead, there is an increased breakdown, in agreement with the study of Nazar

et al.[3] Thus, it appears that even with a high beta-blocking dose, the ability to break down glycogen is not inhibited. The most probable explanation for the increased utilization of carbohydrates is the less available supply of FFA to the exercising muscles. To test whether this holds true, we artificially raised the free fatty acids by giving corn oil and heparin as described elsewhere.[1,6] This increased the FFA in plasma to more than double the normal concentration without any difference in concentration between blocked and unblocked animals. As shown in figure 1, when the animals were fatfed, the glycogen depletion was the same irrespective of the beta-blocking treatment. This indicates that decreased lipolysis after blockade could explain the increased glycogenolysis in the muscles. The findings also support the possibility that, during exercise, glycogen degradation is dependent on muscle contraction, and that blockade of the sympathetic system does not significantly influence the rate of glycogen utilization.

Another mechanism by which muscle can increase carbohydrate utilization is the extraction of more glucose from the blood. Surprisingly, studies performed in humans at a workload of 50 percent of max VO_2 with different beta blockers have not shown any increase in glucose uptake by the working muscles.[6,9] In a recent study, however, we found that with more strenuous exercise (90 percent of max VO_2), the glucose uptake by the exercising legs was increased when the subjects were treated with propranolol (Juhlin-Dannfelt et al., to be published). A further evidence for increased glucose uptake during strenuous exercise is that in the abovementioned study on rats running on a treadmill, blood glucose and liver glycogen concentration were lower in the beta-blocked animals, which suggests an increased glucose uptake by the muscles.

Effect of Training

The stimuli triggering the adaptive changes in skeletal muscle oxidative potential to physical activity are unknown. Much interest has been focused on the catecholamines and the sympathetic nervous sytem. Daily injections of isoproterenol have been shown to give an enzymatic adaptation in the skeletal muscle of the same magnitude as exercise and also to give heart hypertrophy.[17] Chemical sympathectomy with guanethidine sulphate in rats prevents the cardiac hypertrophy normally seen after training,[18] but data presented recently indicate that an intact sympathoadrenal system is not necessary for the increase in skeletal muscle respiratory capacity caused by training.[19]

Thus, it appears that the role for the muscle beta-receptors is still unclear, and an interesting question is whether beta-blockade in patients inhibits or decreases the effect of physical training. It has been argued that the reduced myocardial contractility and heart rate response may limit the exercise conditioning. There are, however, studies showing that in patients with coronary artery disease, physical conditioning can take place. Recently Welton et al.[20] reported results on a group of 20 patients, 9 of whom were treated with propranolol. All patients trained 1 hour, 3 days a week (jogging) for 3 months, and both the blocked and un-blocked subjects increased their calculated maximal oxygen uptake from 25 ml/kg/min to 33/ml/kg/min without any difference between the groups. It can, however, be concluded that further studies are needed to evaluate in detail the effects of beta-blockade on the adaptations induced by training, including cardiac hypertrophy and the increased muscle respiratory capacity.

References

1. Epstein SE, Robinson BF, Kahler RL, Braunwald E: Effects of beta-adrenergic blockade on cardiac response to maximal and submaximal exercise in man. J Clin Invest 44:1745-1753, 1965

2. Ekblom B, Goldbarg AN, Kihlbom A, Astrand P-O: Effects of atropine and propranolol on the oxygen transport system during exercise in man. Scand J Clin Lab Invest 30:35-42, 1972

3. Nazar K, Brzezinska Z, Lyszczara J, Danielewicz-Kotowicz A: Sympathetic control of the utilization of energy substrates during long-term exercise in dogs. Arch Int Physiol Biochim 79:873-879, 1971

4. Nazar K, Brzezinska Z, Kowalski W: Mechanism of impaired capacity for prolonged muscular work following beta-adrenergic blockade in dogs. Pfluegers Arch 336:7278, 1972

5. Jorfeldt L, Wahren J: Leg blood flow during exercise in man. Clin Sci 41:459-473, 1971

6. Trap-Jensen J, Clausen JP, Noer J, Larsen CA, Krogsgaard AR, Christensen NJ: The effect of beta-adrenoceptor blockers on cardiac output, liver blood flow and skeletal muscle blood flow in hypertensive patients. Acta Physiol Scand Suppl 440:30, 1976

7. Juhlin-Dannfelt A, Astrom H: Influence of beta-adrenoceptor blockade on leg blood flow and lactate release in man. Scand J Clin Lab Invest 39:179-183, 1979

8. Muir GG, Chamberlain DA, DeClue DT: Effects of beta-sympathetic blockade on non-esterified fatty acid and carbohydrate metabolism at rest and during exercise. Lancet 1:930-932, 1964

9. Frisk-Holmberg M, Jorfeldt L, Juhlin-Dannfelt A: Influence of long-term anti-hypersensitive alprenolol treatment on hemodynamic and metabolic responses to prolonged exercise in man. Clin Pharm Ther 21:675-684, 1977

10. Astrom H, Frisk-Holmberg M, Juhlin-Dannfelt A: Hemodynamic and metabolic effects of $beta_1$-adrenergic receptor blockade. Stockholm hypertension meeting, 1977, p. 74

11. Hagenfeldt L, Wahren J: Metabolism of free fatty acids and ketone bodies in skeletal muscle. In, Muscle Metabolism During Exercise (Pernow B, Saltin B, eds). New York, Plenum Press, 1971, p 153

12. Drummond GI, Harwood JP, Powell CA: Studies on the activation of phosphorylase in skeletal muscle by contraction and by epinephrine. J Biol Chem 244: 4235-4240, 1969

13. Stull JT, Mayer SE: Regulation of phosphorylase activation in skeletal muscle in vivo. J Biol Chem 246:5716-5723, 1971

14. Issekutz B: Role of beta-adrenergic receptors in mobilization of energy sources in exercising dogs. J Appl Physiol 44:869-876, 1978

15. Richter EA, Galbo H, Christensen NJ: Adrenal medullary control of muscular glycogenolysis in exercising rats. Acta Physiol Scand 105:9-10A, 1979

16. Rennie MJ, Winder WW, Holloszy JO: A sparing effect of increased plasma fatty acids on muscle and liver glycogen content in the exercising rat. Biochem J 156:647-655, 1976

17. Harri MN, Valtola J: Comparison of the effects of physical exercise, cold acclimation and repeated injections of isoprenaline on rat muscle enzymes. 95:391-399, 1975

18. Ostman-Smith I: Prevention of exercise-induced cardiac hypertrophy in rats by chemical sympathectomy (guanethidine treatment). Neuroscience 2: 497-507, 1976

19. Henriksson J, Svedenhag J, Richter EA, Galbo H: Significance of the sympatho-adrenal system for the exercise-induced enzymatic adaptation of skeletal muscle. Acta Physiol Scand 105:38-39A, 1979

20. Welton DE, Squires WG, Hartung H, Miller RR: Effects of chronic beta-adrenergic blockade therapy on exercise training in patients with coronary heart disease. Am J Cardiol 43:399, 1979

SUMMARY: PART 4

Ivar Ringqvist, M.D.

It has been clearly shown that physical training results
in improvement of physical capacity brought about by a
biological adaptation to the physical stress given.
Adaptive reactions occur with endurance training in the
circulatory system, in the nervous system, and in the
skeletal muscles with the augmentation of respiratory
capacity in the muscle cells.

Clausen, Trap-Jensen, and Lassen showed in 1970 that
leg and arm training had little transfer effect on arm
and leg work capacity, respectively. These findings
emphasized that a substantial part of the conditioning
response derives from peripheral adaptation. It also
has implications for the design of cardiac training programs. Many recreational and occupational activities require upper extremity activities. A physical conditioning program should, therefore, include exercises of all
major muscle groups.

Generally, the increase in maximum O_2-uptake capacity
by endurance training results equally from an increase
in cardiac output secondary to a higher stroke volume
and an increase in oxygen extraction in healthy persons.

There are evidences indicating that in patients with
ischemic heart disease, both the increase in maximum
exercise capacity and the increase in endurance during
submaximal exercise are mainly mediated by exercise-
induced adaptations in skeletal muscles. However, we
have to remember that we deal with patients with varying
degrees of coronary heart disease and varying degrees of
impairment of left ventricular function. It seems
probable that many patients with coronary heart disease
also will show adaptations in the heart with physical
training.

Coronary angiography and especially the new noninvasive techniques will help us to define subgroups of patients with ischemic heart disease with different responses to training.

Intermittent claudication is a rather frequent symptom in a population. In man, the prevalence rate increases from 1 percent in the age group 50-54 years to 5 percent in the age group 65-69 years (Framingham Heart Study). The prevalence is lower for women. The natural history of peripheral arterial disease is considered to be benign. However, the mortality rate is about twice the normal, but the patients die from cardiac complications.

Several studies have shown the beneficial effect of physical training in most patients with intermittent claudication. Different causes are suggested to explain the improvement with training, including improved peripheral utilization of oxygen, improved oxidative metabolic capacity, and perhaps improved walking technique, in some cases.

There is a need to further examine the patients who fail to improve from physical training. Their characteristics with regard to the severity of disease of peripheral arteries and especially to the severity of coronary heart disease and the degree of impairment of ventricular function should be defined. Under supervision, more prolonged periods of training or more intensive training could be tried.

It has not been proved that training can prolong the lives of patients with intermittent claudication or stop the progression of the disease. However, if the treatment can improve the walking distance, so that the disease will will be of less hindrance for the patient at work or at his recreational activity, it is a valuable treatment for both the patient and the society.

More and more patients with cardiovascular disease are on beta-blocker therapy. It will, therefore, be of utmost importance to further study the effect of training on central/and peripheral parameters in patients with different types of beta blockers.

Discussion of Chapter by Holloszy

The discussion focused on the relationship between the peripheral effects of training and the central effects. Dr. Bruce stated that the reduction in heart rate and systolic pressure observed after training at submaximum workloads is almost exactly proportional to the reduction in relative aerobic cost or the percentage of the individual's new and higher maximum oxygen uptake. How it is achieved is quite unknown. Dr. Saltin mentioned that the oxidative enzymes in muscles are increased with training out of proportion to the increase in the AV oxygen difference. There is not, however, always a one-to-one relationship between related systems.

The contention that the increase in physical capacity in patients with ischemic heart disease is attained by exercise-induced adaptations in the skeletal muscles and by alterations in the responses of the endocrine and autonomic nervous system, rather than by adaptation of the heart, was opposed. Reference was made to the Duke study, in which noninvasive examinations had shown improved left ventricular function. Dr. Shephard pointed to his material on postmyocardial infarction patients. Most of them had an increase in arterial-venous O_2 extraction during the first 6 months of training, but over the second 6 months, when the patients were able to train harder, a significant increase in the stroke volume was found.

Discussion of Chapter by Saltin

It was pointed out by Dr. Saltin that patients with intermittent claudication can do more work on a bicycle ergometer than they can do on a treadmill. The reason is that they can use the lower part of the leg as a lever if they have the pedal just underneath the foot and not under the toes. There is then little activity in the calf muscles.

There were different opinions about whether the claudication patients increased their mechanical efficiency on walking by training, i.e., the patients learn to walk better. Dr. Saltin pointed to the work by the Goteborg group, which had made a biomechanical study on the patient's walking technique and had not found any difference before and after training. Dr. Ringqvist indicated that it is very difficult to study in an objective way the walking technique, which could explain why no difference was found before and after training.

It was emphasized that at least one-third of the patients with intermittent claudication also had a symptomatic cardiovascular disease. This group of patients requires special attention, with special training programs.

Discussion of Chapter by Juhlin-Dannfelt

The intriguing finding that lactate release is diminished during beta-blocker therapy was discussed. In a recent study by Dr. Bruce et al., a significant reduction was found in ventilation CO_2 and respiratory exchange ratio after beta blockade. The results seemed to be difficult to fit in with the data presented, except in terms of the lowered lactate. Dr. Juhlin-Dannfelt presented data that showed that there is a linear relationship between muscle lactate concentration and lactate release from the working leg, both in unblocked and blocked situations. The question was asked if muscle fatigue is related to accumulation of lactate in muscle during exercise. Dr. Juhlin-Dannfelt's finding in young hypertensives does not support that concept.

PART 5

15

ROLE AND VALUE OF PSYCHOLOGICAL TESTING IN CARDIOVASCULAR REHABILITATION

J. Alan Herd, M.D.

Psychological tests are an important part of the psychological approach to cardiovascular rehabilitation and have the same objectives as medical treatment, which are to a) reduce death and disability from cardiovascular disease, b) improve response to treatment, and c) reduce costs of that treatment.

Psychological techniques can improve outcomes of treatment. They are an inherent part of encouraging patients to exercise regularly, reduce weight, alter diet, take medication, and stop smoking. Psychological techniques are useful in increasing patients' adherence to prescribed programs, to detect and treat depression, and to improve personal and social adjustments following cardiovascular disease. They can reduce costs of treatment through identifying potential problems and by individualizing treatment programs according to objective signs of progress.

Many studies of health and illness in special populations have used psychological tests as predictors of health change. An example of such a study is a 5-year prospective study of air traffic controllers in New York and New England.[1] This study was carried out in collaboration with Drs. Rose, Jenkins, and Hurst at Boston University Medical Center. Four hundred controllers were evaluated according to physical, psychological, and behavioral characteristics and studied prospectively to determine the incidence of illness. Table 1 lists the predictor variables used in the study. Outcome variables included new cases of physical illness, hypertension, psychiatric illness, depression, and anxiety arising during a 3-year period of time. The tests and procedures that included variables most predictive of health change are indicated by numbers at the right of each item.

Table 1: ATC Health Change Study

1.	Socio-Demographic Characteristics Biographical Questionnaire 3

2.	Health History and Health-Related Behavior
	    Medical Questionnaire
	    Medical History
	    Physical Examination 2
	    Smoking, Eating, Drinking Habits

3.	Personality Characteristics
	    California Psychological Inventory 1, 4
	    Jenkins Activity Survey 1, 2, 4
	    MMPI Subscales 1
	    16 Personality Factor Questionnaire
	    ATC Questionnaire 2, 3
	    Interview Ratings 1
	    Psychiatric Status Schedule 1

4.	Marital, Family, and Social Supports ATC Questionnaire 2, 3

5.	Job-Related Characteristics
	    ATC Questionnaire 1, 2, 3, 4, 5
	    Job Description Inventory
	    Leadership Behavior Scale
	    Kavanagh Life Attitude Profile
	    Sociometric Questionnaire 1

6.	Impact of Life Changes 1, 2, 3, 4, 5
	    Review of Life Experiences
	    Schedule of Recent Experiences
	    Life Change Inventory

7.	ATC Workload (Field Measures)
	    Objective Measures
	    Subjective Difficulty Questionnaire

8.	Psychological and Behavioral Measures at Work
	    Profile of Mood States Questionnaire
	    Behavior Rating Scale
	    Subjective Difficulty Questionnaire

9.	Physiological Measures at Work
	    Heart Rate and Blood Pressure 1, 2
	    Plasma Cortisol and Growth Hormone 1

10.	Monthly Health Reports
	    Monthly Health Review
	    Checklist of Symptoms
	    Zung Anxiety and Depression Scales 1

KEY

1 Physical Illness

2 Hypertension

3 Psychiatric Illness

4 Depression

5 Anxiety

Those variables predicting physical illness are marked (1), those predicting hypertension are marked (2), those predicting psychiatric illness are marked (3), those predicting depression are marked (4), and those predicting anxiety are marked (5). It is evident from this list that assessments of performance, health, and morale included not only psychological tests but also interviews, physical examinations, behavioral assessments, and reports by trained observers under field conditions.

Experience with programs for risk factor reduction in healthy subjects also has demonstrated the importance of psychological principles. For a program to be successful, it is necessary to take care of problems, make objective measures of progress, pay attention to what is working and what is not working as soon as possible, and use stringent clinical and social criteria to assess the

significance of progress observed. These principles involve much more than the use of psychological tests.

Psychological tests have several specific uses. They
are designed to evaluate individual aptitudes and abili-
ties (an example is an IQ test), psychomotor skills (an
example is a reaction-time task), and personality characteristics (an example is the Minnesota Multiphasic Personality Inventory). Many tests are based on self-
reports and recollections. They are subjective and
liable to personal bias. Psychomotor skills are tested
using specialized equipment under laboratory conditions.
Performances are subject to confounding factors such as
motivation. Psychological tests form only a part of
complete psychological assessment.

Psychological tests are seldom used alone. They are
remote from actual behavior under natural situations and
they are poor predictors of responses in specific situations. Even direct observation of responses in one
situation provides little basis for predicting responses
in another situation. In addition, results of psychological tests introduce problems of validity and reliability.
They are subject to personal bias and individual interpretation. In a medical or psychological treatment
program, we should decide what behaviors we are trying to
influence and measure those behaviors as directly as
possible. In addition, we should use objective measures
whenever possible.

There are several subjects of specific concern for
cardiovascular rehabilitation programs that include psychological topics. These are adherence to cardiovascular
rehabilitation programs, depression, incomplete recovery
of function, and evaluation of treatment.

Psychological factors govern adherence to prescribed
treatments. They influence the ability of patients to
follow recommendations and to continue in their rehabilitation programs.[2] Severe cardiovascular disease not only
causes physical limitations but also causes depression.[3]
Many patients recovering from acute myocardial infarction
are depressed, and this condition can be detected by psychological assessments.[4] Psychological techniques can
be used to alleviate this condition. Complete recovery
of function may be limited by physical disabilities, but
it also may be limited by psychological and social factors.[5] Evaluating success for a cardiovascular rehabilitation program includes assessing not only recovery of
physical capacity for work but also restoration of normal
daily activities.[6]

Management of patients with depression involves psychological tests, clinical interviews, and behavioral
assessments. Patients in a depressed state also exhibit

a loss of interest in usual activities, an inability to concentrate, psychomotor retardation or agitation, suicidal thinking, weight loss, difficulty sleeping, and feelings of hopelessness. One psychological technique for measuring depression is a self-rating by the patient using a psychological test such as the one developed by Zung.[7] However, self-report scales are influenced by denial and deliberate falsification. Clinical interview improves reliability of diagnosis, especially when the interview is conducted according to a predetermined structure.[8] Even greater reliability in diagnosing depression can be obtained from behavioral assessments of the patient's daily activities interpreted in conjunction with the results of psychological tests and clinical interviews.

A practical approach to treatment of psychological factors includes several components. These components are: determining previous patterns of behavior and levels of function, obtaining baseline measures, prescribing treatment, assessing the program and revising it continually, and evaluating success using objective criteria and quantitative scales.

Figure 1 shows a model of interactions between components. Each patient will respond to a specific situation according to individual goals and expectations.

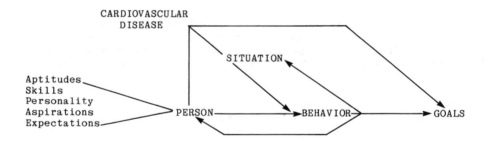

Figure 1

Goals are the desired outcomes of responses. The intensity of efforts to reach goals depends upon expectations that success can be achieved at an acceptable price. Psychological tests, interviews, and behavioral observations provide information about the patient that may be used to predict behaviors. However, behaviors must be observed to be sure the desired goals can be reached. Also, each response affects both the situation and future responses in ways that may change behaviors with time and repetition. Cardiovascular disease affects patient,

214

situation, goals, and outcomes of behavior. All these
interactions should be analyzed and used to develop each
individual treatment program.

Several different techniques are used in treating psychological factors; one is psychological testing. Other
techniques include biographical data (table 2); medical

Table 2:   Biographical Data

Age
Sex
Place of birth
Places of residence
Education
Occupation
Military service
Athletic activities
Hobbies
Social contacts
Religion

Spouse

Age
Background
Education
Occupation

Family

Size
Activities
Contacts

Parents

Family size
Education

---

history and treatment regimen; psychological tests (table
1); interview with patient and spouse or close partner;
contingency contracting; checklist of problems (table 3);
checklist of activities (table 4); diary of activities,
problems, and pleasant events; objective measures of
progress; and clinical and social criteria for success.
Tables 1 to 4 list essential elements of each psychological technique.

Table 3:   Problem Checklist

Somatic complaints (headaches, indigestion, constipation,
   etc.)
Angina pectoris (triggering events, frequency, duration)
Weight gain, diet
Cigarette smoking
Insomnia
Fatigue, tiredness, boredom, inactivity
Anxiety, tension
Depression
Marital relations
Family problems
Financial troubles
Sexual problems
Occupational difficulties

Table 4:   Activities Checklist

Pleasant Events

Problems

Daily Activities
    Sleep, rest, inactivity, reading, TV
    Physical activity, exercise, sports
    Recreation, hobbies, entertainment
    Household, family, errands, chores
    Social contacts, friends and family
       service activities in church, school, community

Work
    Previous work experience
    Special skills, responsibilities
    Hours/day, days/week, months/year
       performance, promotion, awards, recognition salary,
       bonuses, raises, group interactions

Personal
    Sharing, caring, giving
    Sexual activity

Special Concerns
    Diet and eating habits
    Smoking habits
    Medication and special treatment

General Level of Performance
    Establishing priorities
    Scheduling time
    Completing tasks

The strategy for using psychological techniques follows a logical pattern. The steps are 1) initial evaluation, 2) prediction of likelihood for success, 3) recommendations for treatment, and 4) evaluation of progress. Figure 2 shows the steps in chronological sequence.

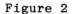Figure 2

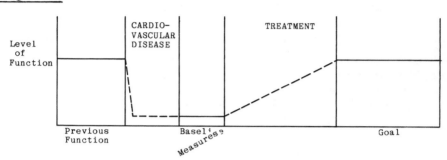

Level of function is affected by cardiovascular disease and must be evaluated according to both previous levels and current levels. This comparison between previous and current levels of function forms a useful basis for establishing goals. However, the goals must be chosen according to aspirations and expectations of the patient. Also, the timetable for reaching goals must be realistic. Previous patterns of behavior and levels of function must be determined and compared with present patterns and levels.

Much of the information required to make assessments can be obtained from the patient; some can be obtained from a spouse or close personal friend; and some information can be obtained from employers, colleagues, and friends. Current patterns of behavior are best assessed using a diary of activities, problems, and pleasant events.[9] Using all of these techniques, the decrements in level of function attributable to cardiovascular disease are determined. A thorough analysis includes considerations of personal characteristics, situation factors, and influences of cardiovascular disease (figure 1).

Predicting the likelihood of success involves analysis of factors influencing adherence to prescribed medical

217

regimens. Factors known to influence adherence to cardiovascular rehabilitation programs[4] are: previous history
of myocardial infarction, cigarette smoking, type A behavior pattern, previous patterns of behavior and levels
of function, involvement of spouse, depression, problems
not easily resolved, and commitment to program. These
factors are listed in table 5. Those patients who are

Table 5: Factors Influencing Adherence

Previous history of myocardial infarction
Cigarette smokers
Type A behavior pattern
Previous patterns of behavior and levels of function
Involvement of spouse or close personal friend
Depression
Problems not easily resolved
Commitment of time, effort, money

---

strongly committed to reasonable goals according to a
realistic timetable, with enthusiastic support of spouse
or close personal friend, are most likely to achieve success in reaching those goals. Also, if you can take care
of problems, patients will perceive value from the program and maintain participation.

Recommendations for treatment involve contingency contracting, methods for recording progress, periodic evaluation, and a process for continual revision according to
progress. Contingency contracting should involve patient
and spouse or a close personal friend. It involves
assessing amount and accuracy of information concerning
medical and psychological conditions, assessing personal
goals and expectations that they can be achieved, lia-
bilities to participation, and evidence of personal commitment. For example, requiring a cash deposit insuring
future performance in meeting a contract assures the
contract will be fulfilled. Payoffs and penalties must
be agreed upon with participation by patient and partner.
All of these conditions should be committed to writing,
with counselor, patient, and partner all signing the
document.

Evaluation of progress should be based upon specific
indicators chosen prospectively. Only three or four indicators should be selected, and their selection should

be based upon reliability of previous patterns of behavior and levels of function as realistic goals for
treatment. Suitable indicators are specific problems,
pleasant events, specific occupational or recreational
activities, and adherence to specific recommendations.

Evaluations should include psychological tests, interviews, checklist of activities, checklist of problems,
diary reports of daily activities, and behavioral assessments by patients, spouse or partner, peers, and trained
observers. When progress is apparent, strategy for
treatment should continue. When progress is not observed, the cardiovascular rehabilitation program should
be revised.

Determining the practical value of a cardiovascular
rehabilitation program requires more than subjective reports from the patient. Even behavioral assessments by
impartial trained observers may not reveal the true
worth of treatment outcomes. Some effort must be made
to assign clinical and social significance to progress.[10]
Demonstrating a statistically significant improvement may
have no practical impact on personal and social adjustments. Clinical and social significance indicates progress that has an impact on daily activities. Whether a
change of clinical or social importance has been achieved
requires analysis of the extent to which change has occurred during treatment and the extent of return towards
previous patterns of behavior or levels of function. The
patient may report that he feels better and functions
better, but if no one can confirm his report, meaningful
progress may not have occurred.

The role and value of psychological assessment in cardiovascular rehabilitation is to focus attention on psychological factors and institute psychological treatments. Psychological techniques provide insight into
previous patterns of behavior and levels of function in
comparison with current measures of performance and capability for improvement. Psychological techniques reveal
goals and expectations of patients and indicate methods
of treatment. Evaluation of progress requires subjective
improvement and evidence of capacity for useful physical
and psychological adaptation. Evaluation also requires
quantitative behavioral assessments. Psychological tests
are an important part of psychological assessment, but
they are not sufficient alone to carry out a successful
cardiovascular rehabilitation program.

References

1. Rose RM, Jenkins CD, Hurst MW: Air Traffic Con-
    troller Health Change Study. FAA Contract No.
    DOT-FA73WA-3211, Boston University, 1978

2. Oldridge NB, Wicks JR, Hanley C, Sutton JR, Jones
    NL: Noncompliance in an exercise rehabilitation
    program for men who have suffered a myocardial
    infarction. Can Med Assoc J 118:361-364, 1978

3. Cassem N, Hackett T: Psychological rehabilitation
    of myocardial infarction patients in the acute
    phase. Heart Lung 2:283-288, 1973

4. Stern MJ, Pascale L, Ackerman A: Life adjustment
    postmyocardial infarction: determining predictive
    variables. Arch Intern Med 137: 1680-1685, 1977

5. Schiller E, Baker J: Return to work after a myo-
    cardial infarction: evaluation of planned rehabili-
    tation and of a predictive rating scale. Med J
    Aust 1:859-862, 1976

6. Naismith LD, Robinson JF, Shaw GB, MacIntyre MMJ:
    Psychological rehabilitation after myocardial in-
    farction. Brit Med J 1:439-442, 1979

7. Zung WWK: A self-rating depression scale. Arch
    Gen Psychiatry 12: 63-70, 1965
8. Zung WWK: The depression status inventory: an ad-
    junct to the self-rating scale. J Clin Psychol 28:
    539-543, 1972

9. Fordyce WE: Behavioral concepts in chronic pain and
    illness. In, Behavioral Management of Anxiety,
    Depression, and Pain (Davidson PO, ed). New York,
    Mazel Press, 1976, p 147

10. Kazdin AE: Assessing the clinical or applied im-
    portance of behavior change through social valida-
    tion. Behav Modif 1:427-451, 1977

16
THE ROLE OF SOCIAL RESOURCES
IN CARDIAC REHABILITATION

Richard T. Smith, Ph.D.

This report is based on a selected review of the literature, with an emphasis on studies that indicate the role
of social resources in the process of recovery along
with studies that provide an empirical base for estima-
ting the magnitude of the cardiovascular disease problem.
Recent reviews and studies have been published which offer more detailed information about social and economic
factors in cardiovascular rehabilitation.[1-4]

Formal intervention systems providing supportive services for the disabled may be necessary elements in the
recovery process, but may not be sufficient by themselves. In addition to these formal systems, informal
social networks may play an important role.[5] The notion
of social support is described by Kaplan and his colleagues in terms of the availability of socially supportive networks in which a "social network includes the
people one communicates with, and links within these
relationships."[6] In examining the crisis of physical
illness, Moos and Tsu point out that the social environ-
ment as a resource includes the relationships of patients
and their families and the social supports in the wider
community, such as friends and clergy.[7]

As sources of support in times of crisis and during
recovery, informal networks may complement the formal intervention system; it is only under extreme conditions,
when the informal network of support fails, that the
individual must rely solely on the formal social network.[8]

Studies have shown that the informal social network,
comprising family, friends and neighbors, constitutes an
important supportive resource for patients recovering

from major health crises. In their study of heart patients, Croog and Levine[4] found that patients reported
extensive use of informal networks, as part of their
"armory of services," in the process of recovery. The
availability and use of kin and non-kin social networks
may be a function of the level of social integration;
"the better integrated the individual, the higher the
degree of assistance he receives."[9] Other evidence presented by Croog and his colleagues suggests that except
for immediate health care, limited reliance is placed on
formal institutions and agencies by individuals recovering from severe illness. A similar finding was noted by
Finlayson and McEwen[10] in their study of heart patients
in Scotland.

Finlayson and McEwen also made similar observations
about the supportive role of informal social networks.
They noted that favorable recovery was associated with
socially supportive networks, in terms of lay help and
consultation, and a wider range of kin and non-kin
sources tended to enhance outcome.[10-11] New and his
colleagues,[12] as well as D'Afflitti and Weitz,[13] found
that significant others, i.e., family and non-kin members, played a supportive role among heart and stroke
patients undergoing recovery and rehabilitation.
Litman,[14] on the other hand, did not find a significant
relationship between family solidarity, i.e., level of
social integration, and favorable rehabilitation response
in his study of orthopedically disabled patients. However, he did find evidence that the family played a supportive role in the patient's convalescence.

With the adult cardiovascularly disabled numbering an
estimated 3.2 million in the U.S. population in 1972,[15]
further investigation of the role of social networks in
the recovery process, especially those outside the domain
of the formal intervention system, seems appropriate.

Some Preliminary Evidence

In a previous study,[16] it was observed that recovery
status was influenced in part by the absence of formal
supportive agents as well as limited use of rehabilitation services. The study population consisted of adults
with primary disabling disease conditions of the circulatory, respiratory, musculoskeletal, and nervous systems.
What is interesting in these findings is the fact that
favorable recovery was associated with an individual's
informal social network, implying that this factor was a
viable source of support. Although the relationship was
not strong, its presence as a determinant does suggest

the importance of informal supportive agents in the process of disability and rehabilitation.

In a related aspect, involvement with the vocational rehabilitation (VR) agency suggests formal intervention support. This should enhance the likelihood of recovery. For the adult disabled, vocational rehabilitation contact generally implies assistance to those with potential capacity, that is, the less severely disabled and younger in age. Therefore, one would expect that contact with the VR agency, as a measure of formal intervention assistance, would further enhance recovery. Those without contact would be expected to show the reverse.

Since VR contact, as an indicator of formal intervention, may be viewed as too limited in scope, and perhaps may not adequately reflect assistance or service received by the adult disabled, an alternate measure was used in the analysis to incorporate the more global nature of rehabilitation services available in the community. As defined, rehabilitation services reportedly refer to all kinds regularly provided by agencies and individuals including hospitals, clinics, physicians, and public agencies such as vocational rehabilitation agencies. This more inclusive measure was examined in relation to recovery status.

As observed in table 1, the results are contrary to conventional expectations. Involvement with rehabilita-

Table 1: Relationship Between Rehabilitation Services and Recovery Status[16]

| Rehabilitation Services | Recovery Status | | | | Total |
| | Low | | High | | |
	No.	Percent	No.	Percent	
Services received	133	(45)	162	(55)	295
None received	186	(43)	247	(57)	433
Total	319	(44)	409	(56)	728

$x^2 = 0.24$, NS.

Base N = 770.

tion services apparently has not had greater effect on recovery. (There is almost complete statistical independence.) More importantly, disabled adults without formal contact with rehabilitation services show a similar rate of recovery to that observed for the disabled with services (57 percent and 55 percent, respectively). Also, about 1 1/2 times as many disabled do not have contact with the rehabilitation service system (59 percent), yet proportionately, the rate of recovery is about the same.

In this particular study, we have observed the effects of other primary agents, especially those from the informal social network, that lend support to the disabled during the process of rehabilitation and recovery. In general, this suggests that the majority of disabled adults received rehabilitation services, of whatever kind, from sources other than the traditional formal intervention system of rehabilitation.

It is suggested that these support systems, comprising informal agents and their social networks as well as other formal nonrehabilitation networks, constitute a viable community resource. Schematically, we can identify four general types of disabled groups in terms of outcome and the provision of rehabilitation services. This is shown in table 2. Rather than the disabled using

Table 2: Rehabilitation Services and Recovery Status: Paradigm of Intervention Modes[20]

Formal Rehabilitation Services	Recovery Status (Outcomes)	
	Recovered	Not Recovered
Received	Intervention Success	Intervention Failure
Not received	Nonintervention Success	Nonintervention Failure

the formal intervention rehabilitation system through agencies and individuals providing such services, as might be commonly expected, the majority of the disabled apparently use other sources of service and seemingly rely on other supportive networks in the community. These cases may be identified as the nonintervention successes in table 2.

There may be limited reliance placed on other formal systems of medical care in the community; a great deal of reliance may be placed on informal social networks, such as the family, associated kin, and friends, as well as on formal, nonrehabilitation agencies and institutions such as unions, employers, and fraternal and religious organizations. Another element may be self-reliance. Both lay roles and informal social networks have been recognized

224

in a recent WHO publication on disability prevention and rehabilitation: "Disabled patients may sometimes by themselves, or with the aid of their families or employers, solve their problems without any external aid."[17]
Furthermore, Martin of Switzerland, in his article on the "active patient," suggests that lay initiatives in health are not inconsequential and, in fact, may make the patient less dependent on the traditional providers.[18] In general, these formal nonrehabilitation agencies and informal social networks seem to constitute the effective support system leading to successful rehabilitation and recovery of the disabled adult.

Magnitude of the Current Cardiovascular Disease Population

Data from existing sources must be used to estimate the extent of rehabilitation effort in the adult population with cardiovascular ("heart") disease. In this instance, information is derived from Social Security Administration (SSA) program data along with recent cross-national survey data. This provides only an indirect assessment of the magnitude of the problem, yet it may be sufficient for purposes of examining the role of social and economic factors in the process of rehabilitation and recovery.

From the 1972 SSA survey of the noninstitutionalized adult population in the U.S., an estimated 15.5 million individuals (ages 20-64) were disabled, of which 3.2 million (21 percent) were identified as disabled due to cardiovascular diseases.[15] Of this latter group, approximately 6 out of 10 (1.9 million; 59 percent) were classified as severely disabled, i.e., unable to work altogether or unable to work regularly.[15]

Using SSA program data for 1972, an estimated 550,000 disabled workers were in current payment status (those allowed disability compensation) because of diseases of the circulatory system (ICDA codes 392-458). This is based on figures showing that about 30 percent of the total number of disabled workers in current payment status (1.8 million) are identified as those with circulatory diseases.[19] (These "allowances" are presumed to be severely disabled, because program criteria of eligibility require a worker to be unable to engage in substantial gainful activity due to a chronic condition.) This represents about 29 percent of the estimated total severely disabled adult population with heart disease in 1972 (550,000/1,900,000).

Based on SSA program data for 1977, about 850,000 adults disabled with circulatory disease conditions were receiving disability compensation (30 percent out of 2.8 million in current payment status). If this represents 29 percent of the total severely disabled with circulatory diseases, the projected number is about 2.9 million. Furthermore, the estimated 2.9 million severely disabled comprises about 59 percent of the total population of adults with circulatory diseases; thus, the overall population of adults with heart disease amounts to approximately 4.9 million.

Extent of the Rehabilitation Effort
In the Recovery Process

From the 1972 SSA survey of disabled adults, 13.3 percent of the heart disease-disabled reported receiving some kind of formal rehabilitation services subsequent to the onset of disablement. In this survey, rehabilitation refers to the services received "because of a health condition which interfered with the individual's ability to work, or do housework;" such services included job counseling and guidance, job training and placement, physical therapy, recreation, training for leisure activities, and special devices.[15] (It is interesting to note that among the severely disabled with heart disease, the proportion receiving rehabilitation services does not differ in any appreciable manner from that observed for the total group: 13.7 percent and 13.3 percent respectively. This is all the more striking given the notion of services needed in relation to severity of disablement; that is, the more severe cases should show higher use than the average.)

For the estimated 4.9 million disabled adults with heart disease, this amounts to 652,000 individuals who have received formal rehabilitation services (table 3). The influence of rehabilitation services as a primary mode of intervention can be assessed in terms of success or recovery. As suggested previously, recovery can be operationally defined as indicative of independence and measured by improvement in health level and social/psychological well-being. Another aspect of formal support through program intervention is that indicated by the percentage of heart disease-disabled receiving Social Security disability insurance compensation. About 29 percent of the total severely disabled with circulatory diseases receive S.S.D.I. benefits, that is, less than one-third receive such support. In fact, this represents only 17.3 percent of the total circulatory disease-disabled population.

Table 3: Rehabilitation Services and Recovery Process:
Estimates of Magnitude of Outcomes for Circulatory
Diseases* (No. in 000's)

Formal Rehabilitation Services	Recovery Status (Outcome)		
	Recovered	Not Recovered	Total
Received	363 (7.4%)	289 (5.9%)	652 (13.3%)
Not received	2,381 (48.6%)	1,867 (38.1%)	4,248 (86.7%)
Total	2,744 (56.0%)	2,156 (44.0%)	4,900 (100.0%)

*Based on estimates for 1977.

Although viewed on a continuum from recovery to lack
of recovery relative to the individual's status following
disability onset, the outcome measure can be dichotomized
for purposes of analysis. As shown in table 3, the estimated 4.9 million heart disease-disabled can be distinguished by their likelihood of recovery. In this instance, previous empirical evidence[16] suggests that
about 56 percent of the disabled will experience improvement and hence can be identified as "recovered." (The
percentage estimate is based on findings of recovery
experiences among adults disabled with major chronic
diseases of the circulatory, respiratory, musculoskeletal,
and nervous systems.) Given these relative indicators
regarding the frequency of rehabilitation intervention
and recovery, the expected cell frequencies for the
adult disabled with heart disease can be estimated as
shown in the table. Also, as previously indicated (table
1), the role of formal rehabilitation services does not
appear to influence recovery; cell frequencies reflect
this statistical independence between formal intervention
and recovery status.

It can be observed that the great majority of heart
disease-disabled do not receive rehabilitation services
(86.7 percent), yet the rate of recovery can be expected
to be proportionately the same as compared to those who
do not receive such services. In addition to health and
psychological influences, what social and economic factors lend support to the disabled's successful recovery?
Empirically, this begs the question: What are the factors that characterize the nonintervention successes in
terms of facilitating a favorable outcome?

It is suggested that the degree of social integration
may be an important determinant in facilitating favorable
outcomes among those chronically disabled with heart disease. Degree of social integration is a function of social resources that takes into account assists and supports derived from primary and secondary groups.[20]
These constitute the effective social support networks
of the individual during the time of crisis and subsequent efforts at coping and adjustment.[1,4,9] The extent
to which supportive social resources are effectively
utilized will in turn result in a favorable effect on
recovery, both with and without formal intervention.
Furthermore, the greater the extent that formal intervention systems co-opt these resources and view them as part
of the support structure of the individual, the greater
the likelihood of recovery.

An individual's social resources may be identified and
operationalized according to the scheme outlined by
Andersen and Newman.[21] This scheme identifies predisposing, enabling, and need factors that are likely to
influence the use of rehabilitation services and eventual
outcome. Factors that predispose the individual to use
services include socio-demographic (e.g., age, sex,
race), structural (e.g., education, occupation), and
beliefs (e.g., values and attitudes toward health and
illness, efficacy of treatment regimens). Enabling factors are those that facilitate an individual's ability
to secure services, and may include family and kin networks, health insurance coverage, compensation benefits,
regular source of care, and access to care. Need factors
identify disease and severity, along with mobility and
activity limitations resulting from the chronic condition.

In examining the role of social resources in the recovery process, one may schematize these sets of factors
in the following manner.

I. **Primary group resources** (informal social system)

    A. **Predisposing factors:**

        1. Personal characteristics (demographic
           attributes such as age, sex, and race
           have social meanings and help define
           the social setting)

        2. Individual structural characteristics (an
           individual's achieved attributes, which
           are brought to the social situation, such
           as educational attainment and occupa-
           tional status)

3. Personal beliefs and attitudes (these factors may influence the definition of the situation, such as internal/external locus of control and beliefs about the efficacy of the role of providers and treatment regimens)

B. Enabling factors:

 1. Family and kin networks (as support systems and as an indicator of level of social integration in primary groups)

 2. Quasi-kin networks (friends and neighbors, work peers, etc., as support systems)

 3. Income and other economic assets (an individual's achieved assets)

II. Secondary group resources (formal social system)

 Enabling factors derived from the following networks:

A. Formal service networks

 1. Public programs (disability insurance, rehabilitation services, social and welfare services)

 2. Private supports (personal physician, private health insurance, other personal health services)

B. Formal social networks (work, fraternal, religious, and other social memberships, including voluntary associations)

Need for rehabilitation services is seen as a determinant in the recovery process, but the measures of need, obtained at onset or immediately post-onset, may be randomized or controlled in the intervention trial.

In conducting a controlled clinical trial with the cardiac disabled for purposes of assessing the efficacy of some particular intervention element, such as physical conditioning exercises, it would seem appropriate to examine the extent to which social resources facilitate recovery and optimize outcome. Figure 1 depicts the hypothesized relationship of rates of success (simulated) for a controlled intervention trial in which rate of recovery is shown to be influenced by level of social resources. The higher the level of social resources, the higher the rate of success, irrespective of intervention.

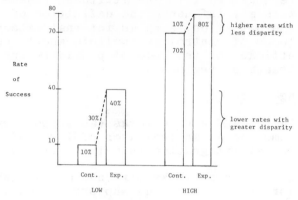

Level of Social Resources*
(*Degree of social integration as measured by extent of
social resources: predisposing and enabling factors.)

Figure 1: Hypothesized Relationship of Rates of Success
for the Heart Disease-Disabled, by Level of Social
Resources, for Clinical (Experimental) and Non-Clinical
(Control) Intervention Groups (Simulated)

This implies that those who possess an armory of social
resources will effectively use them as support mechanisms
in the recovery process. Also, the differential effects
of intervention on success rates between the experimental
and control groups will be less for those with high social resources in comparison with those having low social
resources. Also, this may reflect the observed differential in rate of compliance between those with high versus
low social resources.

This appears to be a feasible working hypothesis that
could be incorporated in a clinical intervention trial
that would take into account the role of socioeconomic
factors in the process of cardiovascular rehabilitation.
More importantly, it may serve to identify the cardiac
disabled who are lacking primary and secondary group
resources and are therefore in need of more structured
supportive services.

In the recovery process, emphasis tends to be placed
on the medical care network as the single most relevant
source of support, to the exclusion of other relevant
sources. However, family and non-kin appear to play a
vital role. This general statement is reflected in the
observation made by Croog and Levine in their study of
heart patients: "Although it is commonly hypothesized
that modern industrial institutions and organizations of
the larger society are taking over many of the roles of
the traditional kin groups, in this . . . study population kin and quasi-kin played important supportive

230

roles."[4] The implication of this finding is evident.
The formal intervention system is complemented by an
"armory of services" that includes links with informal
social networks. In time of crisis and in coping with
severe illness, these social networks constitute important supportive resources for the individual and appear
to be effective in facilitating recovery.

Recognition and use of this extended resource base by
health care providers may be an effective supplemental
tool of therapeutic intervention. As Kaplan and his
colleagues suggest, "modern family medical practice
should include a workgroup of one's 'personal networks'
. . . and consider the possibility of providing or help-
ing provide more functional social networks as an integral
responsibility of the health care system."[6] This suggestion seems aptly suited for the chronically ill and
disabled in society who, in addition to care received
from rehabilitation medicine and health-related service
systems, need to rely on other social networks for
support and long-term care, leading to eventual recovery.

References

1. Croog SH: Social aspects of rehabilitation after
    myocardial infarction: a selective review. In,
    Rehabilitation of the Coronary Patient (Wenger
    NK, Hellerstein HK, eds). New York, John Wiley &
    Sons, 1978

2. Doehrman SR: Psycho-social aspects of recovery from
    coronary heart disease: a review. Soc Sci Med
    11:199, 1977

3. Monteiro LM: Cardiac patient rehabilitation. So-
    cial aspects of recovery. New York, Springer
    Verlag, 1979

4. Croog SH, Levine S: The heart patient recovers.
    Social and psychological factors. New York, Human
    Services Press, 1977

5. McKinlay JB: Some approaches and problems in the
    study of the use of services. An overview. J
    Health Soc Behav 13:115, 1972

6. Kaplan BH, Cassel JC, Gore, S: Social support and
    health. Med Care (suppl) 15:47-58, 1977

7. Moos RH, Tsu VD: The crisis of physical illness.
    An overview. In, Coping with Physical Illness
    (Moos RH, ed). New York, Plenum, 1977

8. Susser MW, Watson W: Sociology in medicine.
    London, Oxford Press, 1971

9. Croog SH, Lipson A, Levine S: Help patterns in
    severe illness: the roles of kin network, non-family
    resources, and institutions. J Marr Family 34:32,
    1972

10. Finlayson A, McEwen J: Coronary heart disease and
    patterns of living. New York, Prodist, 1977

11. Finlayson A: Social networks as coping resources.
    Lay help and consultation patterns used by women
    in husbands' post-infarction career. Soc Sci Med
    19:97, 1976

12. New PK, et al: The support structure of heart and
    stroke patients: a study of significant others in
    patients' rehabilitation. Soc Sci Med 2:185, 1968

13. D'Afflitti JG, Weitz GW: Rehabilitating the stroke
    patient through patient-family groups. In, Coping
    with Physical Illness (Moos RH, ed). New York,
    Plenum, 1977

14. Litman TJ: The family and physical rehabilitation.
    J Chron Dis 19:211, 1966

15. Treitel R: Rehabilitation of disabled adults, 1972.
    Social security disability survey 1972: disabled
    and non-disabled adults. Report No. 3, 1977

16. Smith RT: Rehabilitation of the disabled. Interna-
    tional Rehab Med, 1(2) (table 4), 1979

17. World Health Organization. Disability prevention
    and rehabilitation. 29th World Health Assembly.
    A 29/INF Doc/1, 1976

18. Martin JF: The active patient: a necessary develop-
    ment. WHO Chronicle 32:51, 1978

19. Unpublished SSA tabular data, 1978

20. Smith RT: Disability and the recovery process.
    Role of social networks. Chapter 12. In, Patients,
    Physicians, and Illness (3rd ed) (Jaco EG, ed).
    New York, Free Press, 1979

21. Anderson R, Newman J: Societal and individual de-
    terminants of medical care utilization in the United
    States. Milbank Mem Fund Q 51:95, 1973

SUMMARY: PART 5

Albert Oberman, M.D.

Psychological factors play a key role in the successful rehabilitation of a patient following myocardial infarction. Persistent anxiety and depression[1,2] as well as myocardial damage can result in failure to return to work, resume social activites, remain free of symptoms, or otherwise make satisfactory life adjustments. Patients with minimal coronary disease and more than adequate left ventricular function may remain disabled due to unresolved psychosocial conflicts. Progress in cardiovascular rehabilitation depends in large part on a better understanding of a variety of nonmedical problems after myocardial infarction. Some determinants of successful long-term outcome, as reflected by return to functional levels and lifestyle seen prior to infarction, include the family structure and personal relationships, attitudes of personal physicians and employers, and social support within the community.

Toward this end, Dr. Herd described the role and value of psychological testing and Dr. Smith reviewed social and and economic factors relating to cardiovascular rehabilitation. Dr. Herd incorporates psychological techniques to promote health-related behavior, including adherence to treatment, and to improve the outcome of treatment. Specific psychological concerns for rehabilitation programs consist of adherence to treatment, depression, incomplete recovery of function, and treatment evaluation. A pragmatic approach to treatment of psychological factors involves a comprehensive evaluation of the patients' problems, ascertaining that goals are realistic, documenting previous behavior patterns, and assessing functional capacity as compared to previous levels. Besides psychological testing, a variety of techniques can be used for behavioral evaluations, such as interviews, contingency contracting, checklist of problems and activities, diaries, objective measures of progress, and finally, clinical and social criteria for success.

Psychological tests by themselves are remote from natural behavior and consequently cannot predict specific responses in various situations. Furthermore, they are developed for individuals with psychopathology and may be neither appropriate nor sensitive enough for more general populations. Some useful tests from the standpoint of assessing adherence and depression are the Jenkins Activity Scales (type A behavior) and the Jung Index, respectively. Using psychometrics to assess outcome is futile--the evaluation must include an index of what an individual is doing as well as what he says he does or how he says he feels. Patients may tell us how great they feel, but quality of life must be translated into some objective index or measure. The best way to determine whether a patient is showing improvement may be actual performance, both on and off the job, or related variables such as frequency of hospitalization or utilization of physician services. Efforts must be made to define clinical and social progress during recovery in order to gauge and modify psychological attempts at intervention during this period.

Dr. Smith focused on the informal social network, comprising family, friends, and neighbors, as the most important resource for patients recovering from major medical problems. Only when this support fails does the individual rely on the more formal social facilities. Contrary to expectations, formal rehabilitative services exert little influence on recovery. Smith estimated, on the basis of Social Security Administration data for 1977, that about 850,000 adults with circulatory disease were receiving disability compensation. Based on this estimate, the projected total number of severely disabled adults with circulatory disease is about 2.9 million. He noted that about 13 percent of patients received formal rehabilitation services, yet their rehabilitation success rate was no higher than for those who did not receive such services.

Smith categorized the informal social system by 1) predisposing factors--age, sex, race, education, occupation, and health beliefs--and 2) enabling factors-- family, friends, and neighbor networks plus economic assets. He outlined the formal social system as secondary group resources, consisting of service networks, such as public programs and private supports (e.g., health insurance and personal physician), and social networks, such as memberships in social and fraternal organizations. The higher the level of those social resources, the higher the rate of recovery success, as measured by return to work, nonlimitation of activity, source of income, and physician supervision, thus obviating the need for any formal intervention. Those individuals who need more structured social services tend to be those who have limited informal and community resources and also may not have the necessary self-reliance. It appears that social support mechanisms, motivation, and self-image determine outcome as much as, or more than, clinical considerations. Medical practitioners must recognize and take advantage of informal social networks, in addition to the more formal service system, to provide much-needed support for a more complete recovery.

Few would dispute the importance of psychological factors in effecting optimal long-term recovery from myocardial infarction. Much can be gained from careful psychosocial assessment and consideration of the impact of these factors on rehabilitation. Drs. Herd and Smith have outlined important considerations toward implementing appropriate psychosocial services. However, physicians lack the necessary validated psychosocial tools for both therapeutic evaluation and intervention. Unless such techniques can be further developed and made available to practitioners, psychosocial stresses will continue to serve as barriers to rehabilitation.

References

1. Hackett TP, Cassem NH: Psychologic Aspects of Rehabilitation After Myocardial Infarction. In, Rehabilitation of the Coronary Patient (Wenger NK, Hellerstein HK, eds). New York, John Wiley & Sons, 1978, p 243

2. Needs and Opportunities for Rehabilitating the Coronary Heart Disease Patient: Report of the Task Force on Cardiovascular Rehabilitation of the National Heart and Lung Institute, Public Health Service, U.S. Department of Health, Education, and Welfare, December 15, 1974

PART 6

17

CARDIAC REHABILITATION: CURRENT PHYSICIAN ATTITUDES

Charles K. Francis, M.D.

Cardiac rehabilitation has become widely accepted and is
considered desirable in the management of patients with
coronary as well as other forms of cardiac diseases. In
order to better understand their attitudes, expectations,
and level of knowledge concerning physical conditioning
and rehabilitation of cardiac patients, a questionnaire
was mailed to 250 physicians in the greater Hartford,
Connecticut, area.

The physician names comprised the mailing list of the
American Heart Association, Greater Hartford Chapter. A
total of 60 physicians (24 percent) responded to the
questionnaire. Ten questionnaires were considered unsuitable for tabulation. The majority of the unsuitable
responses were from physicians who had retired or whose
practices were limited to the pediatric age group. Of
those returning the questionnaire, 40 percent actually
had done exercise stress testing in their practices.

Respondents referred patients to rehabilitation and
physical conditioning programs for a variety of reasons
(table 1). The most commonly stated purpose for outpatient referral was physical conditioning and rehabilitation following a myocardial infarction. Other indications, in decreasing order of frequency, were stable
angina, obesity, lipid disorders, and family history of
coronary disease. The recommendation that patients
engage in prescribed physical conditioning activities
following myocardial infarction was made by 82 percent
of the respondents. Exercise testing as a screening
procedure was most commonly recommended for postmyocardial infarction patients (table 2).

Table 1:   Reasons for Outpatient Physical Conditioning

Stable Angina	37
Family History	28
Lipid Disorders	29
Obesity	33
Post-MI	41

Table 2:   Exercise Test As Screening Procedure

Stable Angina	29
Family History	20
Lipid Disorders	16
Obesity	1
Post-MI	33
Atypical Chest Pain	19
Before Exercise Program	7
Routine, Over Age 40	0

Routine stress testing for persons over 40 years of age was not felt to be a suitable practice by any respondent. Exercise testing as a screening procedure in asymptomatic patients with chest pain of uncertain etiology and/or stable angina was the next most commonly selected reason for ordering an exercise test. Family history, lipid disorders, and atypical chest pain were also frequently selected reasons for ordering a screening exercise test.

The duration of stay following myocardial infarction related directly to future rehabilitation and physical

conditioning programs. The preferred length of stay
following myocardial infarction was 12 days (table 3).

Table 3: Length of Hospital Stay

Hospital Days Post-MI	
8 days	5
12 days	37
16 days	5
20 days	1
Exercise Test Post-MI	
Discharge	5
2 weeks	1
4 weeks	6
6 weeks	7
8 weeks	4
12 weeks	4

The duration of stay varied from 8 days to 20 days, with
the greatest number of respondents selecting a total stay
(postmyocardial infarction) of 12 days. Opinions regarding the appropriate interval for exercise stress
testing postinfarction was diverse, ranging from testing
at discharge to testing at 12 weeks.

The current popularity of physical conditioning and
exercise may in some degree be explained by the attitudes
of physicians regarding the effects of inpatient cardiac
rehabilitation and physical conditioning (table 4). In
contrast to previously held fears of aneurysm formation,
reinfarction, and/or dysrhythmias resulting from exercise
and rehabilitation in postinfarction patients, these complications were not felt by our respondents to be increased by inpatient physical conditioning and rehabilitation. Inpatient physical conditioning and rehabilitation programs were felt to have no effect on mortality

by 30 (60 percent) of the respondents.

Table 4: Physician Attitudes about Inpatient Physical
Conditioning and Rehabilitation

Inpatient Program	Increase	Decrease	No Change	Unknown
Mortality	2	10	30	8
Morbidity	3	25	15	7
Reinfarction	2	5	30	13
Aneurysms	5	0	39	6
Dysrhythmia	5	3	34	8
Contractility	17	1	26	6
CAD progression	0	10	28	12
Health costs	12	14	14	10
Physician control	19	7	15	9
Return to work	30	1	11	9

By contrast, however, 25 (50 percent) felt that rehabilitation would decrease morbidity significantly.
Interestingly, 15 (30 percent) felt morbidity was unchanged. A surprising divergence of opinion was noted
regarding the effect of rehabilitation on myocardial
contractility. Contractility was felt to be increased
by cardiac rehabilitation in 17 (34 percent) of the
responses, whereas 26 (52 percent) felt contractility
would remain unchanged. In spite of increasing recommendations of cardiac rehabilitation for patients with coronary artery disease, 28 (56 percent) felt progression of
coronary disease would remain unaffected by such rehabilitation. Significantly, 12 (24 percent) had no
opinion and 10 (20 percent) felt progression of the
disease would be reduced.

The impact of physical conditioning and cardiac rehabilitation on health costs is a major concern in planning future programs and expanding current activities.
There was no clear consensus regarding the impact of
inpatient cardiac rehabilitation by our respondents: 12
(24 percent) felt health costs would increase; 14 (28
percent), that they would decrease; and 14 (28 percent),
that they would remain unchanged. Ten (20 percent)
had no opinion. The ability of physicians to control
their patients' therapeutic regimens was felt to be increased by 19 respondents (38 percent), in contrast to
15 (30 percent) who felt there would be no change. The

242

major impact of inpatient cardiac rehabilitation was felt by 30 respondents (60 percent) to be an increased rate of return to work.

Outpatient cardiac rehabilitation and conditioning programs were considered more effective than inpatient programs in several significant areas. Outpatient programs in general were felt to be of greater usefulness in reducing morbidity and mortality, with 28 (56 percent) expecting deaths would be reduced and 36 (72 percent) expecting morbidity would be lessened. The danger of reinfarction was also felt by 25 (50 percent) to be lessened, whereas 21 (42 percent) felt there would be no change. Significantly, 38 (75 percent) felt that aneurysm formation would not be affected significantly, whereas 29 (58 percent) felt that dysrhythmias would not be affected at all (table 5).

Table 5: Physician Attitudes about Outpatient Physical Conditioning and Rehabilitation

Outpatient Program	Increase	Decrease	No Change	Unknown
Mortality	0	28	19	3
Morbidity	1	36	10	3
Reinfarction	0	25	21	4
Aneurysms	5	2	38	5
Dysrhythmia	2	11	29	8
Contractility	26	1	15	8
CAD Progression	0	24	14	12
Health Costs	11	28	4	7
Physician Control	26	5	14	5
Return to Work	38	0	6	6

In spite of a lack of substantial data indicating a beneficial effect on contractility, 26 (53 percent) indicated that contractility would be increased by physical conditioning and rehabilitation in patients postinfarction. A beneficial effect was expected by 24 (48 percent) respondents, who felt that progression of coronary disease would be decreased, whereas 14 (28 percent) thought there would be no change. Health costs were expected to decrease by 28 (56 percent) respondents. Increased physician control was expected by 26 (52 percent), and 38 (76 percent) felt that the rate of return to work would be increased by their patients' participation in an outpatient cardiac rehabilitation program.

In comparing attitudes concerning outpatient versus inpatient programs, the beneficial effects of outpatient programs appear to outweigh those of inpatient in the opinion of our respondents (table 6).

Table 6: Physician Attitudes about Physical Conditioning and Rehabilitation--Inpatient and Outpatient Programs

	Increase		Decrease		No Change		Unknown	
	I	O	I	O	I	O	I	O
Mortality	2(4%)	0(0%)	10(20%)	28(56%)	30(60%)	19(38%)	8(16%)	3(6%)
Morbidity	3(6%)	1(2%)	25(50%)	36(72%)	15(30%)	10(20%)	7(14%)	5(6%)
Reinfarction	2(4%)	0(0%)	5(10%)	25(50%)	30(60%)	21(42%)	13(26%)	4(8%)
Aneurysm	5(10%)	5(10%)	0(0%)	2(4%)	39(78%)	38(76%)	6(12%)	5(10%)
Dysrhythmia	5(10%)	2(4%)	3(6%)	11(22%)	34(68%)	29(58%)	8(11%)	8(16%)
Contractility	17(34%)	26(52%)	1(2%)	1(2%)	26(52%)	15(30%)	6(12%)	8(16%)
CAD Regression	0(0%)	0(0%)	10(20%)	14(48%)	28(56%)	14(28%)	12(24%)	12(24%)
Health Costs	12(24%)	11(22%)	14(28%)	28(56%)	14(28%)	4(8%)	10(20%)	7(14%)
Physician Control	19(38%)	26(52%)	7(14%)	5(10%)	15(30%)	14(28%)	9(18%)	5(10%)
Return to Work	30(60%)	38(76%)	1(2%)	0(0%)	11(22%)	6(12%)	9(18%)	6(12%)

I = inpatient; O = outpatient.

Although drawn from a relatively small survey, these data provide some indication of physician attitudes concerning physical conditioning and rehabilitation for patients with cardiovascular disease. The use of exercise testing in the immediate postinfarction period, either before discharge or soon after, appears to have become accepted as a useful means of assessing prognosis and determining further treatment. Most of the respondents to this survey have shortened the duration of hospital stay following myocardial infarction to approximately 12 days, with some physicians sending patients home as early as 8 days.

The opinion of the Ad Hoc Committee on duration of hospitalization that a 9- to 14-day duration of stay following myocardial infarction should suffice in "complicated, completed acute myocardial infarction" seems to have been accepted in clinical practice.[1] Exercise testing has become a commonly used screening procedure in evaluating patients following infarction as well as part of standard diagnostic procedures in evaluating chest pain of uncertain etiology. Routine stress testing of asymptomatic individuals without other significant risk factors was not commonplace among the physicians responding to our survey.

244

Concerns about increasing morbidity, mortality, and complications were relatively rare. Few respondents felt that either inpatient or outpatient cardiac rehabilitation and physical conditioning would result in increased rates of reinfarction, aneurysm, or dysrhythmias. The expectation of increased ventricular contractility resulting from physical conditioning was common with both inpatient and outpatient programs, even though the effect of exercise on contractility remains moot.

The expectations of the clinicians responding to our survey may indeed be justified by recent evidence suggesting a role of the Frank-Starling mechanism in improving left ventricular function with severe exercise in experimental subjects.[2] The most generally accepted benefit of physical conditioning and rehabilitation in patients with cardiovascular disease was an increased ability to return to work among such patients. Additionally, anticipated reduction in health costs and increased maintenance of physician control of patients following myocardial infarction (presumably resulting in enhanced compliance with medical therapy and reduction in future risk for coronary events) was also common.

The concerns addressed in the questionnaire were diverse but provide some indication of clinician attitudes in a medium-sized northeastern community concerning exercise testing, physical conditioning, and cardiac rehabilitation. The wide spectrum of attitudes and levels of related knowledge reflected by the responses suggests that more factual and objective information concerning the effects of cardiac rehabilitation is necessary among clinicians using exercise testing as well as among those referring patients to cardiac rehabilitation programs.

Many of the assumptions and expectations made by these clinical practitioners lack objective documentation. Most striking of these was the presumption that physical conditioning and rehabilitation will enhance contractility. Although many of the respondents had definite opinions about the dangers and benefits of cardiac rehabilitation, there was general agreement that additional investigative studies on the effects of in-hospital and post-hospital rehabilitation were necessary (table 7).

Table 7: Physical Conditioning and Rehabilitation

Further Study Needed By:	
Random multicenter trial	33
Clinical research centers	19
Community hospital	16
Medical school	13

References

1. Swann HJC, Blackburn HW, DeSanctis R, Frommer PL, Hurst JW, Paul O, Rapaport E, Wallace A, Weinberg S: Duration of hospitalization in "uncomplicated completed acute myocardial infarction." Am J Cardiol 37:413-419, 1976

2. Weiss JL, Weisfeldt ML, Mason SJ, Garrison JB, Livengood SV, Fortuin NJ: Evidence of Frank-Starling effect in man during severe semisupine exercise. Circulation 59:655-661, 1979

246

18
THE NATIONAL EXERCISE AND
HEART DISEASE PROJECT

John Naughton, M.D.

The National Exercise and Heart Disease Project (NEHDP)
is a five-center clinical trial sponsored by the Rehabilitation Services Administration (now the National Institute for Handicapped Research of the Department of Education) of the Department of Health, Education, and
Welfare to determine the effects of medically prescribed, regularly performed physical activity on selected outcomes of cardiac rehabilitation. The project was
funded initially in June, 1972, with the prospect that
it would be a definitive clinical trial in which up to
4,300 myocardial infarction subjects would be studied in
a randomized manner for as few as 5 and as many as 7
years.

   However, funding limitations and a major agency policy
change made in June 1973 mandated a study on a much smaller scale. The project investigators recognized from
the outset that the crucial question of the effect of

Others contributing to this chapter are: Albert Oberman,
M.D., Glenda Barnes, R.N., Del Eggert, M.Ed., Edgar
Charles, Ph.D., Herman Hellerstein, M.D., Jorge Insua,
M.D., Chaim Yoran, M.D., Paul Fardy, Ph.D., Barry A.
Franklin, Ph.D., Charles Gilbert, M.D., Daniel Lee
Blessing, M.S., Barbara Johnson, R.N., Patrick Gorman,
M.D., Margie LaVille, R.N., Marcia Everett, M.S., Alan
Barry, Ph.D., James Daly, M.D.,* John Satirsky, M.D.,
William Marley, Ph.D., Lawrence Shaw, A.M., Patricia
Cleary, M.S., Jorge Rios, M.D., Melvin Stern, M.D.,
Donald Paup, Ph.D., Dan Bogarty, Patricia Kavanaugh,
Sarah Schlesselman, M.S., John LaRosa, M.D., and
Barbara E. Moriarty.

*Deceased December 1979.

exercise on mortality and morbidity probably could not be answered by the trial but that other important questions, concerning exercise testing, the rehabilitation process, and the effects of physical activity on selected physiological, psychosocial, and vocational outcomes, might be answerable.

Therefore, the investigators agreed to pursue a more limited, five-center trial. The centers were located in Washington, D.C.; Philadelphia, Pennsylvania; Cleveland, Ohio; Atlanta, Georgia; and Birmingham, Alabama. The work was coordinated through a centralized coordinating center, with a biostatistical center located in Bethesda, Maryland and an electrocardiography center in Washington, D.C.

Project Design

First Evaluation: The project was designed as a randomized trial in which male survivors of one or more myocardial infarctions were referred to each collaborating center for an initial evaluation (E_1). This evaluation included a complete history and physical examination, standard chest X-ray; 12-lead plus Frank X, Y, and Z lead ECG, recorded at supine rest; measurement of plasma cholesterol and triglyceride levels; pulmonary function testing; and completion of a number of psychosocial questionnaires, including the Minnesota Multiphasic Personality Inventory (MMPI). Plasma HDL was measured on subjects from two of the centers. The spouses completed the Katz Adjustment Scale (KAS). Each subject performed a standardized, multistage exercise test (MSET) on a motordrive treadmill.

PREP: Subjects who satisfactorily completed E_1 were admitted to a 6-week prerandomization exercise program (PREP), in which each subject was required to attend 14 of 18 consecutively scheduled sessions within a period of 6 weeks before proceeding on to the second evaluation (E_2). A total of 12 weeks was allowed for the completion of this requirement. PREP was designed as a program in which patients would become familiar with the activity requirements of the randomized treatment phase of the project, then decide whether to continue in the study, and in which adherence would be promoted. It was thought from the outset that this would permit subjects to drop out early without damaging the randomization process; the likelihood of dropout during the actual trial would thus be reduced. Since the investigators did not wish to dilute the effects of therapy, PREP was conducted as a low-level, nonconditioning program in which subjects' peak activity heart rates were not permitted to exceed

248

The NTG subjects were treated as controls. Project staff were advised not to counsel the NTG subjects about physical activity nor to encourage an activity not considered a part of their daily routine. These subjects were reevaluated on the same schedule as the ETG subjects.

Duration of Followup: All subjects were followed for at least 2 1/2 years, and 70 percent were followed for 3 years.

Subject Characteristics

A total of 931 men were referred for study. Of these, 651 completed the requirements of E_1, PREP, and E_2; 323 were assigned to ETG and 328 to NTG. The subjects ranged in age from 30 to 64 years, with a mean of 51.8 years. Six percent were under age 40, 78 percent were aged 40 to 59, and 16 percent were aged 60 to 64.

Seventeen percent had sustained more than one myocardial infarction (MI). Forty-seven percent were earning $20,000 or more per year. Ninety-four percent were white. Twenty percent entered NEHDP from 2 to 6 months, 37 percent from 7 to 12 months, and 43 percent from 13 to 36 months post-MI.

The mean measurements and standard deviations for the 651 subjects were: height, 174 ± 8.1 cm; weight, 79 ± 10.7 kg; body fat, 20 ± 3.4 percent; plasma cholesterol, 223.2 ± 53.7 mg/100 ml; plasma triglycerides, 179 ± 158.2 mg/100 ml; total forced expiratory ventilation, 3.7 ± 0.8 l; and timed forced expiratory ventilation, 2.9 ± 0.6 l (78 percent).

Selected Observations

The NEHDP clinical trial was completed on May 31, 1979. Data analysis will consume the major portion of a project year, and a final report together with appropriate publications will be submitted on behalf of the project staff and the subjects. Only selected observations are available, therefore, for this report. Among them are observations on the desirability of an 85 percent versus a 100 percent APHR-limited exercise test, the effects of 6 weeks of low-level physical activity on performance capacity, the prognostic value of an exercise test, and the effect of long-term training on performance capacity.

85 percent of the peak heart rate level reached at the first MSET. For those subjects who reached 85 percent of their age-predicted heart rate (APHR), this meant that the PREP exercise heart rate could not exceed 72 percent of their APHR. In other words, the lower the activity heart rate during PREP, the better.

PREP sessions were conducted three times a week. Subjects exercised on six different machines: arm-wheel, hand crank, rowing machine, treadmill, bicycle ergometer, and steps. Each performed at each station for 4 minutes. Heart rate level was controlled with a cardiotachometer, to which the patient was attached via hard-wire cable. Each activity was interspersed by 2 minutes of rest.

Second Evaluation: A second evaluation (E_2) was completed at the conclusion of PREP. This evaluation was comparable to E_1, except that during the second exercise test, subjects were permitted to work to the 100 percent age-predicted heart rate (APHR) level in the absence of symptoms or abnormal signs instead of being arbitrarily terminated at 85 percent APHR, as was the situation for E_1.

Randomization: The subjects were randomly assigned by the biostatistical center to either an exercise treatment group (ETG) or a nontreatment group (NTG). Of the 931 subjects initially referred for study, 651 completed the requirements of E_1, PREP, and E_2, and of these, 323 were assigned to ETC and 328 to NTG. Once assigned, subjects were considered members of their group until the completion of the project, whether they adhered to the treatment assignment, had surgery, or dropped out.

Post-Randomization Program: Subjects assigned to ETG were given an updated physical activity prescription at each evaluation. For the first 8 weeks post-randomization (post-R), they met in the facilities used for PREP. The activity was conducted in the same manner, except that each subject was permitted to work to 85 percent of his peak heart rate as measured at the second MSET. All subjects were reevaluated 8 weeks post-R and at 6-month intervals post-R until the completion of the trial.

The ETG subjects were entered in a gymnasium program after the first post-R evaluation. This program also met three times a week, but the format included games, walking-jogging, calisthenics, and swimming. It was supervised by project staff, but no attempt was made to monitor the exercising heart rates with the precision and accuracy employed during PREP and the first 8-week period post-R.

Observations on an 85 percent heart rate-limited exercise test
versus a 100 percent limited procedure

The 651 subjects performed two MSET's approximately 7
weeks apart. The procedures were identical, except that
the first was terminated at 85 percent of the subjects'
APHR in the absence of abnormal symptoms or signs and
the second at 100 percent. The investigators selected
this methodology for the first MSET because they were uncertain how many early-recovery patients would be referred for study and to ensure patient safety. In addition, had the full-scale study been implemented as initially visualized, this methodology would have promoted
quality control.

Any of eight warning codes was used to terminate an
MSET. These were: symptoms, physical signs, ischemic
ST-T changes in the ECG, ventricular arrhythmias, systolic blood pressure in excess of 225 mmHg, diastolic
blood pressure increase of 20 mmHg or more above resting
level, and subjective determination that the subject
could proceed no further.

The findings from the two MSET's quite clearly established the 100 percent APHR procedure as the preferred
approach. In the first MSET, 54 percent of the 651 subjects reached 85 percent of their APHR in the absence of
overt cardiovascular abnormality. At the second MSET,
only 15 percent of the subjects reached 100 percent.
Thus, the 100 percent APHR precipitated or aggravated
more overt cardiovascular limitation and, at the same
time, provided an improved determinant of the actual
level of aerobic work capacity. Since both procedures
were performed without precipitating a major cardiovascular event, both were judged as safe.

Since exercise testing has never before been applied
to such a large population sample in a consistently
rigorous manner by a group of collaborating centers, the
data provide meaningful standards concerning levels of
aerobic work capacity among patients. For the 100 percent MSET, the mean aerobic work capacity was 7.9 MET's.
A relationship of work capacity to endpoints was observed; subjects capable of reaching the higher heart
rate levels had a mean work capacity of 9.5 MET's, compared to a capacity of 7.6 MET's for symptom-limited
subjects and 7.2 MET's for sign-limited subjects. Although the latter two values do not differ significantly,
the sign-limited subjects were consistently lower in
performance capacity across all ages.

The second MSET provided valuable physiological observations concerning the adaptation of systolic blood pressure and heart rate to graded levels of exercise. These
parameters were evaluated in relation to level of work

capacity attained, reasons for stopping their MSET, and age. For purposes of these analyses, the endpoints were grouped into three classifications: symptom-limited (overt symptoms or a subjective sense that subject could proceed no further), sign-limited (ECG changes, physical signs, blood blood pressure abnormality), and heart rate-limited (100 percent of subject's APHR reached in the absence of symptoms or signs).

The findings indicated a close correlation between level of work capacity achieved and level of peak heart rate reached. In other words, the lower the aerobic threshold, the lower the mean peak heart rate response. This relationship was confirmed by the finding of lower peak heart rates but higher mean peak heart rates among the symptom-limited and sign-limited subjects. As expected, the mean peak heart rate decreased with age, in part because of the employment of the "100 percent of APHR" criteria. On the other hand, mean peak systolic blood was not related to these variables in the same way. Mean peak systolic pressure did not differ significantly according to reason for stopping MSET or by virtue of age. Only for the subjects with significantly reduced aerobic thresholds, i.e., $\leq$ 6 MET's, was the mean peak value significantly lower than for the other variables.

The above findings suggest that of the two variables, heart rate is the principal determinant used for meeting the myocardial oxygen requirements of exercise in MI subjects. Thus, changes in double project (SBP x HR x 10^{-2}) among these variables reflect mainly the contribution of heart rate and not of SBP.

The effects of PREP

The findings from the second MSET were confounded by the slight change in protocol, and therefore, a special analysis was required to discern the relative contribution of this protocol change and of the low-level physical conditioning program to the relative differences in aerobic threshold in results from the second procedure.

A major part of this analysis was accomplished by measuring second-MSET changes in heart rate and systolic blood pressure at the same workload at which the highest heart rate was measured for each subject in the first procedure. The findings indicated that at the second MSET the subjects attained (after conditioning) a mean aerobic threshold 0.57 + .04 MET's higher, the mean peak heart rate decreased 9.$\overline{2}$ bpm, and the mean peak systolic blood pressure decreased 7.4 mmHg. The absolute mean difference in work capacity between the two protocols

252

was 1.6 MET's. The mean difference ascribed to the methodological change approximated 1.0 MET, and to physical conditioning, 0.57 MET's.

These findings indicated clearly that as few as 14 exercise sessions, even though of a low degree of intensity, were sufficient to produce a significant cardiovascular training effect.

Prognostic value of exercise testing

The results recorded at 100 percent APHR were evaluated to determine whether subsequent mortality and morbidity bore any relationship to selected outcomes. A total of 39 deaths and 40 recurrent MI's were documented for the 36 months following this exercise test. The relationship of mortality and morbidity to level of aerobic capacity, peak systolic blood pressure, peak heart rate, and ST-T segment depression on the Frank lead X were determined.

The findings indicated a significant relationship of mortality to all four variables, with the highest relationship being to level of aerobic capacity and peak systolic blood pressure. Subjects with an aerobic threshold of 6 MET's or less had 4.5 times the mortality rate experienced by subjects with aerobic capacity levels of 7 MET's or more. The event rate for subjects with peak systolic blood pressures of 140 mm Hg or less was three times that of subjects who exceeded 140 mm Hg. Subjects who did not exceed 85 percent of their APHR had twice the mortality experience of those who exceeded the 85 percent APHR level, and subjects who had 1.0 mm (0.1 mV) or more of ST-T depression on lead X with exercise had 2.5 times the mortality experience of those who did not. Morbidity bore no relationship to any of these variables.

Since some investigators have emphasized the significance of a low peak heart rate response to exercise, the data were analyzed in terms of high (> 7 MET's) and low (≤ 6 MET's) work capacity levels and by degree of peak heart rate achieved, i.e., < 85 percent or > 85 percent of the APHR. The findings indicated no significant relationship of level between mean peak heart rate reached and mortality which suggests that aerobic capacity, not level of peak heart rate, is the most important determinant of future fatal events. Thus, the concept of chronotropic incompetence, the inability to achieve a high heart rate response, obviously deserves further critical physiological and clinical appraisal.

On the other hand, the relationship of a low peak systolic blood pressure to subsequent mortality was almost
equal in importance to level of aerobic capacity. These
findings suggest that the above subjects have probably
lost the greatest amount of myocardial integrity of all
subjects tested and thus were not able to increase their
cardiac outputs to equal the level of external work
imposed during the testing.

The above findings do not invalidate the concept that
cardiac subjects as a group cannot attain the same peak
heart rate thresholds observed in presumably heathy subjects. Rather, they confirm the findings of other investigators and lend credence to the concept of "heart rate
impairment" (HRI). For those 555 subjects incapable of
reaching 100 percent of their APHR, the mean degree of
HRI was 17.5 percent; for subjects of 6 MET's or less,
it was 24.7 percent, and for subjects of 7 MET's or more
13.9 percent. The data were analyzed by age, and it was
determined unequivocally that HRI relates to level of
aerobic capacity achieved, not to age.

The effects of long-term training

The post-randomization MSET's were used to determine
changes in the ETG and NTG subjects. At randomization,
ETG subjects had a mean aerobic capacity of 7.8 MET's and
NTG subjects, 8.0 MET's. Eight weeks later, the ETG subjects had experienced a significant increase to 8.6
MET's, while the NTG subjects remained essentially unchanged.

From 6 months to 1 year post-R, the ETG subjects experienced an additional modest increase in aerobic
capacity only, while the NTG subjects declined slightly
in aerobic capacity. From 1 year post-R to the end of
the trial, both groups lost aerobic capacity, with ETG
subjects experiencing a more dramatic change than NTG
subjects from 18 to 24 months post-R.

These findings indicate that the trial was effective
in inducing a physiological training effect, but that it
was not sustained throughout the course of the trial.
These data are being evaluated to determine whether factors such as compliance and adherence are related or
whether factors of selection for training (sick subjects,
no; well subjects, yes) explain the difference.

Summary and Conclusions

The National Exercise and Heart Disease Project was designed to determine the effects of medically prescribed, regularly performed physical activity on selected outcomes of the cardiac rehabilitation process. In many respects, it is a feasibility trial that has provided data and experiences that may prove invaluable should a larger-scale, definitive trial of exercise and heart disease be necessary. In size and scope, it was comparable to the trials reported by Sanne in Sweden and investigators in Ontario. In contrast to those trials, it attempted to deal more specifically with a range of rehabilitation issues, including the value of the stress test, exercise testing methodology, and physiological, psychosocial, and vocational outcomes.

The investigators have, at the very least, established the feasibility of conducting such a trial. The cooperation of the subjects was good, and each collaborating center staff remained intact throughout the course of the trial. The findings have provided new insights into testing methodology, the prognostic value of an exercise test, the physiological adaptation to low-level and high-level physical conditioning, and the long-term training process. The definitive results, in terms of mortality and morbidity. will be available in mid-1980.

References

1. Naughton J et al: The National Exercise and Heart Disease Project: development, recruitment, and implementation. Cardiovascular Clinics, Albert N Brest, Editor-in-Chief. Exercise and The Heart (Nanette Kass Wenger, ed) 1978, p 205

2. Naughton J et al: The National Exercise and Heart Disease Project: the pre-randomization exercise program. Report no. 2 (Gallette PM, ed). Cardiology 63:352-367 S. Karger, Publishers, 1978

3. Naughton J: The National Exercise and Heart Disease Project. Heart disease and rehabilitation (Pollock ML, Schmidt DH, eds). Houghton Mifflin Professional Publishers, Medical Div, 1979, p 330

4. The Project Staff: Adaptation to sub-maximal and near-maximal multiple stage exercise tests (in preparation)

5. The Project Staff: The physiological effects of a low-level physical activity program of six weeks duration (in preparation)

6. The Project Staff: Predictors of mortality from a near-maximal exercise test (in preparation)

19
EVALUATION OF EARLIER STUDIES: EUROPE

Veikko Kallio, M.D.

Short-term physical exercise programs after acute myocardial infarction (AMI) are routinely applied in many
European countries although the emphasis varies from
place to place, even in a given country. The programs
differ in intensity, timing, duration, etc., depending on
the aims of the program. A generally accepted objective
is to readjust patients to normal life after AMI.

Most earlier studies of the effects of physical exercise have focused on its physiological effects in carefully selected and relatively small patient groups.
These studies have given valuable information and produced no evidence of any harmful effects. They have,
however, not given a definite answer on how to properly
implement physical exercise in the rehabilitation programs, and particularly what is the role of physical
training in secondary prevention after AMI. A few controlled studies on the feasibility and effects of physical training in AMI patients performed in Scandinavia
have elucidated some of the problems connected with a
long-term physical training program.[2-6] In this paper I
shall summarize the design and main results of these
studies. I shall also present some data of a WHO-coordinated study on rehabilitation and comprehensive secondary prevention in patients after AMI, which has been per-
ormed in 23 centers of 14 European countries and 1 center
in Israel. The results of this study are, unfortunately,
not yet available, but I shall briefly report on some
results from the two participating centers in Finland.

Controlled Feasibility Studies on the Effects
of Physical Exercise

The study of Kentala[2] was aimed at clarifying the
feasibility of supervised physical training in an unselected series of AMI patients with special emphasis on
the significance of physical fitness and supervised physical training for the resumption of work and the prognosis. The basic series consisted of 298 consecutively
hospitalized male AMI patients under 65 years. At admission, the patients were divided into a control group and
a training group according to their years of birth. After exclusion of deaths (24 in the control group and 21
in the training group), and patients with uncertain diagnosis and those living outside the area, there remained
81 patients in the control group and 77 in the training
group. Despite some minor differences in risk characteristics, the groups can be considered to be comparable
for a study on the feasibility of physical rehabilitation.

The length of hospital stay was similar in both
groups. To ensure that the patients were given similar
basic treatment during the followup period, they attended
the outpatient department once a month for examination.
The training program of the exercise group was started 6
to 8 weeks after the infarction. It consisted of two,
and later three, training sessions weekly. The intensity
of the 20-minute exertion phase was regulated to keep the
working heart-rate about 10 beats below the rate tolerated at the maximal load in the exercise test. A physiotherapist supervised the training program at the department of physical medicine. A physician and resuscitation
equipment were always available. In addition to the hospital program, the patients in the training group were
given written advice to increase their physical activity
at home.

Supervised physical training with an attendance rate
of 70 percent or more was feasible in only about 1/5 of
these unselected infarction patients. The attendance
rate fell clearly during the second half of the training
period (figure 1). Main reasons for low attendance rate
or nonparticipation are given in table 1. In addition
to the patients who participated in the supervised training sessions there were another 16 patients maintaining
physical activity at training level on their own accord.
After a year, there were 11 patients in the control group
maintaining physical activity at full training level.

As expected from the poor feasibility of supervised
physical training and contamination of the control group,
no differences between the control and training groups in

Table 1:   Main Reasons For Low Attendance Rate
           or Nonparticipation

	Number of Patients	
	2 - 5 months	6 - 12 months
Work	13	17
Difficult journey	7	7
Severe angina	5	7
No wish to train	4	7
Severe pulmonary failure	4	4
Severe cardiac failure	3	3
Self training	2	4
Other reasons	6	13
Total	44/73	62/72

Kentala, 1972.

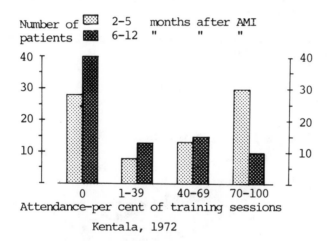

Kentala, 1972

Figure 1

physical working capacity, measured 5 and 12 months after
AMI, were seen.   Resumption of work, morbidity, and mortality were also similar in both groups.   The patients
with an attendance rate of 70 percent or more in supervised physical training improved their physical working
capacity significantly more than other members of the
training group.   One recurrent AMI occurred during the
training sessions.   Locomotor complications were few.

A Swedish trial[4,6] studied whether supervised physical
training could reduce death and nonfatal reinfarctions in
a nonselected series of patients after AMI.   The study
comprised all patients born in 1913 or later who had MI's
during a period in 1968-1970 and were discharged alive

from the hospital. The 313 patients were randomly allocated to a control group and a physical training group.
All patients were treated at a special postmyocardial infarction clinic in order to standardize the followup and
treatment with the exception of the training program.
Twenty seven percent of the patients originally allocated
to the training group had to be excluded before the beginning of the training program. The main reasons for
exclusion were cardiac contraindications and poor cooperation or practical difficulties.

The training program was started 3 months after the
AMI. It consisted of three 1/2-hour training sessions a
week, supervised by a physiotherapist, with a physican in
a nearby room. The highest training heart rate in patients with no evident sign of cardiac limitation averaged
144 beats/min which was 80 percent of their heart rate
increasing capacity (highest heart rate at the maximal
exercise test minus heart rate at rest). The corresponding heart rate for patients limited by angina pectoris
was 136 beats/min.

The dropout rate during the 4-year period of training
is illustrated in figure 2.

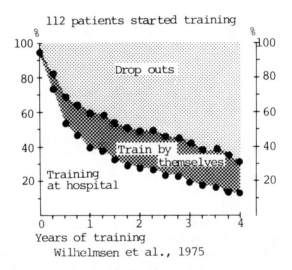

Wilhelmsen et al., 1975

Figure 2

At the followup one year after AMI, only 39 percent of
those who started training were training at the hospital
and an additional 29 percent trained at home. Out of
10,026 training sessions there was one reinfarction
started with ventricular fibrillation. The patient was
successfully resuscitated and was working full time after
the incident.

The physical working capacity, determined one year after AMI, was significantly greater in the training group
and particularly in two subgroups of the training subjects, namely in those who stopped the exercise test because of fatigue or angina pectoris, than in corresponding control group patients. The perceived exertion at a
certain workload had also decreased significantly compared with the control group. During the followup period
of 4 years, 18 percent (28 patients) died in the experimental group and 22 percent (35 patients) in the control
group. The percentages of nonfatal reinfarctions were
16 and 18, respectively. These differences were not significant. Although the high dropout rate might be one
reason for the negative results of this trial, the authors suggest that physical training does not deserve
high priority in the secondary prevention of AMI.

Another Finnish study by Palatsi[3] was designed to determine feasibility and effects of physical rehabilitation based on spontaneous home-training. Subjects with
severe motor invalidity, psychiatric cases, and patients
with severe decompensated heart failure were excluded.
The final series consisted of 180 training subjects, 143
men and 37 women; and 200 controls, 166 men and 34 women
under 65 years.

The first training session took place 2.5 months after
AMI. A physiotherapist conducted the exercise and the
whole session was supervised by a physician. The program
lasted for about 30 minutes and the patients were in-
structed to perform it at home every day. The subjects
came for supervised sessions once a month. Between these
sessions they trained at home, making notes of their own
activity. The program was continued for 12 months. The
interval training technique was aimed toward bringing up
the pulse rate to at least 70 percent of the maximum age-
predicted pulse rate.

The subjects in the control group were also seen once
a month and an ergometer exercise test was performed. No
special program was organized for these patients.

After one year, 51 percent of the men and 73 percent
of the women reported that they were exercising 6 to 7
days of the week. Fifteen percent of the men and 14 percent of the women did an insignificant amount of calis-
thenic exercises.

No significant differences were noted in the symptoms
of coronary disease, clinical findings, and physical
working capacity (PWC 130) between the training subjects
and the controls. A symptom-limited maximal exercise
test was performed on a sample of the subjects. According to the results of this test the training subjects

seemed to improve their physical working capacity more than the controls.

Patients in the training group had a somewhat lower incidence of reinfarctions and coronary mortality than the controls after a followup period of an average of 31.5 months in training subjects and 26.5 months in the controls. During this followup period there were 18 (10 percent) coronary deaths in the training group and 28 (14 percent) in the control group. During the followup period, 21 trainers (11.7 percent) and 29 controls (14.5 percent) suffered a reinfarction. These differences were not, however, statistically significant.

A feasibility study on the effects of physical training with maximum intensity after AMI was recently published in Denmark.[5] The material was selected from a consecutive series of patients--men under 60 years old with a confirmed AMI admitted to the hospital. Apart from age the following exclusion criteria were used: a previous AMI, angina pectoris, heart failure, hypertension, valvular disease, diabetes requiring drug treatment, other complicating diseases, or other factors, which would prevent the patients from taking part in a physical training program. The final series included 54 patients who were randomly allocated in a control group and a training group. During the followup, an additional 8 patients from the control group and 12 patients from the training group were excluded (poor motivation, recurring AMI, etc.). After the above exclusions there were 19 patients in the control group and 15 in the training group. The groups were comparable as regards some basic data at the beginning of the study.

The first exercise test (maximal) was performed during the third week after the AMI. The followup investigations were made 3, 6, and 13 months after discharge from the hospital.

The training program was started one month after discharge. The program was carried out as interval training for 60 minutes twice a week during 12 months. The program consisted of 5- to 6-minute periods of high intensity exercise alternating with 4- to 6-minute periods of lower intensity. During high intensity intervals, the patients were pushed to their subjective maximum.

The work capacity of the training patients was increased by 101 percent compared to a 28 percent average increase in the control group. One episode of cardiac arrest occurred after several months of uncomplicated but irregular training. The incident took place during light calisthenics. The patient was successfully resuscitated.

Conclusions Based on the
Feasibility Studies

The controlled feasibility studies referred to above have produced no evidence of any harmful effects of supervised or advised training. Long-term supervised training was feasible in selected AMI-patients only, including those, particularly, who could train to fatigue and who were well motivated. Even maximum intensity training programs could be used in selected patients. Advised home-training connected with monthly supervised sessions was not sufficient to increase the physical working capacity more than was accomplished through routine medical treatment.

The studies referred to above have not given a definite answer on the secondary preventive effects of an intensive long-term physical training program. This kind of study, although indicated and desirable, would be connected with several difficulties due to poor compliance with the program, contamination of the control group, etc.

The WHO-Coordinated Study

Rehabilitation has been an integral component in the long-term program of the WHO Regional Office for Europe for the prevention and control of major cardiovascular diseases. In several expert working groups convened by the European Office of WHO since 1967, it was considered necessary to further develop particularly the rehabilitation of patients after AMI. Discussions were held about the possibility of designing a long-term project for studying the effects of several years of continuous physical training on mortality and morbidity. Such a study was not, however, considered realistic mainly for the following reasons:

1) High drop-out rate shown in some earlier feasibility studies;

2) Difficulties in collecting the number of patients sufficient for statistically significant results to be obtained;

3) The rapidly changing attitudes on physical training of AMI-patients, exercise programs being applied routinely for coronary patients;

4) There was a need to develop a more comprehensive
    approach, including an efficient application of
    up-to-date knowledge, to postinfarction patients.

As a result of several years' preparatory work a WHO-
coordinated study on rehabilitation and comprehensive
secondary prevention in patients after AMI was designed
(WHO 1973). The study was started in 1973 and ended in
1978.

The study was aimed at assessing the effectiveness of
comprehensive rehabilitative and preventive programs in
reducing recurrent AMI and cardiovascular disease mortality and at contributing to the early physical, psychosocial, and vocational rehabilitation of these patients.
It was designed as a prospective controlled study to be
carried out at a national level but with an attempt to
pool as much information as possible at the international
level.

Male patients under the age of 65 years with definite
acute myocardial infarction, treated in hospital, were
admitted to the study. Because physical training was
just a part of the intervention, no exclusion criteria
from the study were applied.

The following randomization procedures were used:
randomization of individual patients; randomization of
areas, such as hospitals, factories, or communities; and
arbitrary designation of hospitals, etc., as controls.

It was realized that the last-mentioned procedure
might induce a bias in the selection of the material.
The first two methods were thus to be preferred.

All the patients were to be followed up for 2 years
after the onset of AMI. The followup period was, however, prolonged to 3 years for statistical reasons.

After discharge from the hospital, patients in the
control group received further treatment and advice as
routinely provided by the existing system of medical
care in the community. The program in the intervention
group consisted of optimal medical treatment, diet (reduction of overweight and hyperlipidemias), control of
hypertension, anti-smoking education, physical activity
programs, and psychosocial and vocational measures.

The intervention measures were to be applied according
to the best knowledge in each individual center. Concerning physical activation of the patients it was recommended that every center make arrangements for either
supervised or recommended programs (or both), adapted to
the needs of individual patients. For patients with
contraindications for regular physical training, advice

was to be given about physical habits. Special emphasis
in these patients was to be given to the other rehabilitative measures.

Emphasis was given to standardization of evaluation
methods and measurements. The WHO Regional Lipid Standardization Laboratory in Prague provided serum samples
and technical assistance to improve the performance of
local laboratories. An ECG-coding laboratory was set up
in Budapest to assist in coding of ECG's. The rehabilitation clinic in Waldkirch, Freiburg im Breisgau (FRG),
acted as a center for advice on heart size measurement.
A central laboratory for advice on exercise tests for
the study was set up in Brussels. No standardized tests
for psychological evaluation could be adopted by the
working group. It was, however, recognized that research
in this field should be stimulated and the Central Institute of Cardiology in Moscow acted as a center for advice
on psychological problems.

The main endpoints were death (cardiovascular disease
death and other cause of death), morbidity (reinfarction,
cardiac failure, thromboembolism, stroke, other), and
number of hospitalizations and number of days spent in
the hospital (for cardiovascular disease and for other
reasons).

Physical working capacity, changes in the quality of
life, and reduction in ischemic heart disease risk characteristics (e.g., serum cholesterol, blood pressure,
smoking, etc.) were used as additional evaluation criteria.

Although the study was not planned as an international, standardized, controlled clinical trial, pooling of
some data is possible. Preliminary data show that in
spite of different randomization procedures leading to a
difference in the final number of intervention and control patients (table 2), the distribution of patients

Table 2: Randomization of Individual Patients and
Hospitals or Areas in the Intervention and Control Groups

| Group | Randomization of | | Total |
	individual patients	hospital or areas	
I	833	797	1630
C	815	673	1488
Total	1648	1470	3118
Centers	15	9	24

WHO-coordinated study.

with various risk factors (previous infarction, cerebro-
vascular accident, diabetes mellitus, cigarette smoking,
cholesterol above 250 mg/dl) appeared to be equal in
both groups. History of arterial hypertension was somewhat more common in the control group. The complications
during the hospital phase were almost equally distributed
in both groups.

The percentages of patients participating in supervised or nonsupervised physical training at 1-, 2-, and
3-year checkups are shown in table 3. The high percent-

Table 3: The Percentages of Patients Participating in
Supervised or Nonsupervised Physical Training at 1-, 2-,
and 3-Year Checkups

Participation in Physical Training	Group	At review		
		1 yr	2 yrs	3 yrs
Supervised (%)	I	44.8	37.3	30.4
	C	1.7	3.4	2.1
Nonsupervised (%)	I	79.4	77.0	72.8
	C	61.5	58.3	58.9

WHO-coordinated study.

ages of the control patients participating in nonsupervised training indicate that physical exercise is being
routinely recommended for the patients after AMI.

The WHO-Coordinated Study in Finland

I shall, with the kind permission of the other responsible Finnish investigators, Dr. Hamalainen of Turku,
and Prof. Hakkila and Dr. Luurila of Helsinki, briefly
report on some combined results from two Finnish centers
participating in the WHO-coordinated study. The patient
material consisted of 375 consecutive subjects under 65
years who had been treated at the hospital for verified
acute myocardial infarction. At dismissal, the patients
were randomly allocated in an intervention group and a
control group (figures 3 and 4). No significant differences existed between the groups as regards the previous
history, complications, and clinical findings at dismissal from the hospital.

The program of the intervention group was designed according to the principles presented earlier in this paper.

266

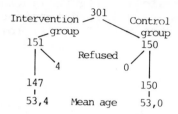

301 < 65 years male AMI-patients

Figure 3

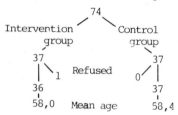

74 < 65 years female AMI-patients

Figure 4

The patients of the control group were treated at their own initiative making use of routine medical services.

The cumulative percentages of total and coronary mortality, sudden deaths, and patients with nonfatal reinfarctions are shown in table 4.

Table 4:   The Cumulative Percentages of Total and Coronary Mortality, Sudden Deaths, and Patients With Nonfatal Reinfarctions

	I	C	
Total mortality	21.8	29.9	$p < 0.10$
CHD-mortality	18.6	29.4	$p = 0.02$
- sudden deaths	5.8	14.4	$p < 0.01$
Non-fatal reinfarctions	18.1	11.2	$p < 0.10$

Serum cholesterol (figure 5) and triglyceride values (figure 6) and both systolic (figure 7) and diastolic (figure 8) blood pressure values determined at 1-, 2-, and 3-year followups were significantly lower in the in-

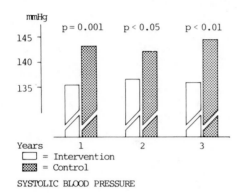

SYSTOLIC BLOOD PRESSURE

Figure 5

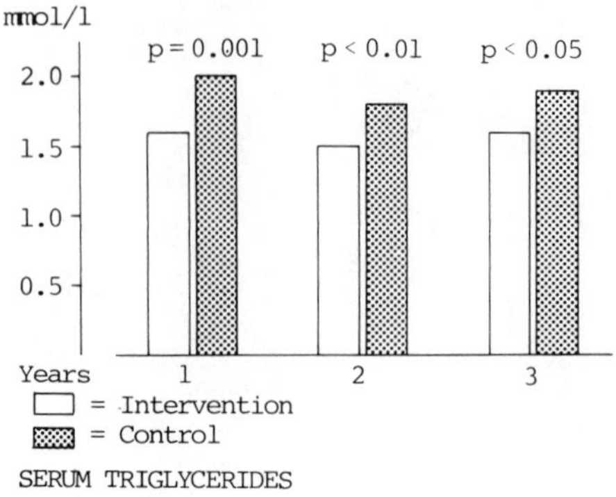

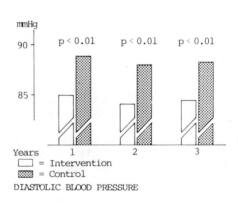

SERUM TRIGLYCERIDES

Figure 6

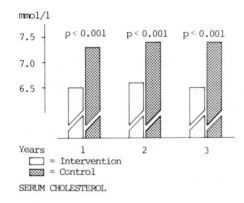

SERUM CHOLESTEROL

Figure 7

DIASTOLIC BLOOD PRESSURE

Figure 8

tervention group than in controls. No significant differences existed in the physical working capacity measured at the yearly checkups (figure 9).

Cardiac failure during the hospital phase seemed to have grave prognostic significance in both the intervention and control groups. The cumulative 3-year coronary mortality of patients with either marked or mild cardiac failure at hospital phase was about 46 percent in both groups.

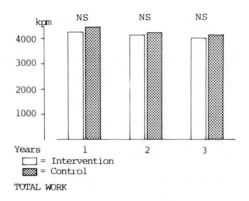

Figure 9

The mortality of patients with first AMI and those with malignant arrhythmias under hospital phase was, however, somewhat lower in the intervention group than in controls.

The results of the two Finnish centers suggest that patients with AMI would benefit from an organized comprehensive rehabilitation and intervention program. No single factor responsible for this effect could be pinpointed.

Summary

It can be concluded that on the basis of the feasibility studies performed in patients after AMI, a physical training program even with maximum intensity is feasible, but the dropout rate is relatively high even during the first 6 months. No significant secondary preventive effect of physical training has been shown in the studies referred to in this paper.

A comprehensive multifactorial rehabilitation and prevention study coordinated by the European Office of WHO is at present being analyzed, and the results are expected to be available during 1980.

The results of the Finnish centers participating in the WHO-coordinated study suggest that it is possible to reduce the CHD mortality and especially the number of sudden deaths after AMI by an early multifactorial intervention program.

References

1. Kallio V, Hamalainen H, Luurila O, Hakkila J: Multi-factorial intervention programme on patients after myocardial infarction. Trans Eur Soc Cardiol 1:070, 1979

2. Kentala E: Physical fitness and feasibility of physical rehabilitation after myocardial infarction in men of working age. Ann Clin Res, suppl, 1972

3. Palatsi I: Feasibility of physical training after myocardial infarction and its effect on return to work, morbidity and mortality. Acta Med Scand, suppl 599, 1976

4. Sanne H: Exercise tolerance and physical training of non-selected patients after myocardial infarction. Acta Med Scand, suppl 551, 1973

5. Saunamaki KI: Feasibility and effect of physical training with maximum intensity in men after acute myocardial infarction. Scand J Rehab Med 10:155-162, 1978

6. Wilhelmsen L, Sanne H, Elmfeldt D, Grimby G, Tibblin G, Wedel H: A controlled trial of physical training after myocardial infarction. Prev Med 4:491-508, 1975

7. World Health Organization: Evaluation of comprehensive rehabilitative and preventive programmes for patients after acute myocardial infarction. Report of two working groups, Prague 1971 and Moscow 1972. WHO Regional Office for Europe, Copenhagen, 1973

20
EVALUATION OF EARLIER STUDIES: CANADA

Roy J. Shephard, M.D., Ph.D.

To those who are eager to begin the experiment, it may
seem a simple matter to conduct a trial testing the value
of exercise rehabilitation in patients with clinically
recognized heart disease. Several million dollars later
the problems inherent in such an undertaking begin to
emerge. It thus seems appropriate to discuss some of
the difficulties that have surfaced in previous U.S.,[1]
Swedish,[2] Finnish,[3] and Canadian[4] investigations, not in
a spirit of flagellation, but rather as a means to the
rational design of a definitive study.

This chapter will review in particular experience
gained from the Southern Ontario Multicentre Exercise-
Heart Trial. This study has followed cohorts of patients
with myocardial infarction for periods of 4 years. It
has involved 7 universities and 12 principal and 7 associate investigators. The information presented is necessarily preliminary, most subjects having participated in
the investigation for about 2 years at the time of data

The views presented in this chapter are the personal opinions of the author.

Principal investigators of the Southern Ontario Multi-
Centre Exercise-Heart Trial are G. Andrew, C. Buck, D.
Cunningham, N. Jones, T. Kavanagh, N. Oldridge, J.C.
Parker, P. Rechnitzer, S. Sangal, R.J. Shephard, J.
Sutton, and M. Yuhasz.

Associate investigators are F. Berkman, P. Demers, R.
Fowles, P. Milos, B. Morton, P. Taylor, and R. Tinning.
The project is supported by a grant from the Ontario
Ministry of Health, Project 263.

review. The conclusions drawn are the personal viewpoint of the author.

Criteria of Ischemic Heart Disease

The basis for entry to the study could theoretically include the appearance of significant exercise-induced ST-sequential depression, angina, or a frank myocardial infarction. We decided that the first two characteristics showed too much day-to-day variation for our purpose. Entry to the Canadian study was thus 3 to 12 months after a clear-cut infarction, documented by two of three criteria: (1) a typical history of chest discomfort, (2) serial ECG changes typical of transmural or subendocardial infarction, and (3) a typical evolution of serum glutamic oxaloacetic transaminase or creatine-phosphokinase readings (peak values >60 and 40 units respectively).

Four of the seven centers were not directly affiliated with hospitals, so that their subjects were referred by cooperating physicians. In the remaining three centers, principal investigators were associated with university teaching hospitals, and could recruit patients directly from the cardiac wards. Taking account of the population of the seven regions, final recruitment figures were 0.14/1000 for referred subjects, and 0.52/1000 with more direct hospital recruitment.

Initially, we chose to exclude patients older than 54 years and those with heart failure, a diastolic pressure greater than 110 mm Hg, insulin dependent diabetes, orthopedic disabilities that would limit progressive exercise, and significant airway obstruction ($FEV_{1.0}/FVC$ <60 percent). The consent of the family physician to participate was mandatory. Patients were required to complete an informed consent form that (1) agreed to randomization, testing procedures and frequencies, and the proposed exercise regimens, (2) acknowledged the slight risks of the experiment, and (3) explained the option of withdrawal at any point in the study.

Following recruitment and clinical examination, volunteers were allocated in a stratified random fashion[4] to either a high intensity endurance exercise regimen (HIE group) or a low intensity homeopathic program of recreational exercise (LIE group). In this way, we hoped to distinguish any benefits of vigorous exercise from the more subtle advantages of participation in a health-oriented group. Stratification of disease (table 1) was in terms of angina, hypertension (blood pressure greater than 160 mm Hg systolic or 95 mm Hg diastolic), blue or

272

white collar occupation, and personality type (Rosenman "A" or "B").

Table 1: Stratification of Participants in the Southern Ontario Exercise-Heart Trial

| | | Personality Type A | | Personality Type B | | |
		Normotensive	Hypertensive	Normotensive	Hypertensive	Total
Angina	Blue collar employment	50	12	38	9	109
	White collar employment	78	16	26	4	124
No angina	Blue collar employment	113	25	59	14	211
	White collar employment	199	36	65	7	307
Total		400	89	188	34	751

Considerations of Sample Size

In any clinical trial of a potential treatment for chronic disease, the sample size depends upon (1) the endpoints selected, (2) the length of the observation period, (3) the estimated attrition rate, (4) the dimensions of the therapeutic effect, and (5) the power of statistical proof that is sought.

For the present purpose, endpoints could conceivably have included the development of symptoms or signs of ischemic heart disease. However, we preferred to adopt the objective endpoints of reinfarction, death, or defection from the study. Four years of observation was suggested as a length of time allowing for a possibly delayed therapeutic effect, while minimizing the logistical problems of an extended study. Given our specific entry criteria, we estimated that 23 percent of our sample would sustain a reinfarction over a 4-year period.[5] We further assumed that a 50 percent reduction of the reinfarction rate would have substantial clinical significance and that the cumulative dropout rate would not exceed 25 percent from either high or low intensity exercise groups. From these assumptions, we calculated that a sample size of 450 would give us an 80 percent chance of demonstrating an effect at the 0.05 level of probability. Later, it was decided to increase the sample size to 750 (table 2); this would allow a dropout rate of 35 percent, while reducing the beta error from 20 percent to 10 percent. As an ethical safeguard, it was decided that the experiment should be halted if either the initial hypothesis were proven or if it were demonstrated that the proportion of reinfarctions in the high intensity exercise group exceeded 67 percent of the sample. The supervising statistician thus monitored events by the technique of sequential analysis.[6]

Table 2: Critical Assumptions of the Southern Ontario Exercise-Heart Trial

---

90% chance of showing an exercise effect, P $\leq$ 0.05

Population

244 High intensity exercise

244 Low intensity exercise (control)

262 Dropouts (35% of each group)

Recurrences

23% Over 4 years in low intensity exercise

11.5% Over 4 years in high intensity exercise

Severity of Myocardial Infarction

There are currently a number of systems for rating the severity of infarction and the subsequent disturbance of left ventricular function:

(1) A clinical score based on age, heart size, pulmonary congestion, and previous ischemia;[7]

(2) Sophisticated mathematical analyses of ECG and vector-cardiographic changes;

(3) Integration of serial increases in serum enzyme readings;

(4) Analysis of left ventricular contractility by echocardiography, angiography, rheocardiography, or analysis of systolic time intervals;[8]

274

(5) Analysis of left ventricular perfusion by angiography or scintigraphy.[9]

However, when many centers are involved it becomes a formidable task to ensure that patients are rated comparably in the various cooperating institutions. Partly for this reason, we have attempted no global definition of severity of disease in our sample, although reinfarction rates will be examined in terms of the individual stratifying variables (table 3).

Table 3: Status of 751 Participants in Southern Ontario Multicentre Trial-- Preliminary Data Obtained After an Average of 20 Months Observation

Current Status	Group		
	HIE	LIE	Total
Active	187	178	365
Dropout	158	143	301
Fatal reinfarction	6	6	12
Nonfatal reinfarction	24	14	38
Died (other cause)		1	1
Completed the study	11	23	34
Total	386	365	751

HIE = high intensity exercise; LIE = low intensity exercise.

When organizing an exercise trial for the post-coronary population, there is inevitably a suspicion that the least severely-diseased patients will be recruited. Even if the trial is controlled, the results will then have generality only for patients with minor degrees of infarction. Angina of effort was initially present in 233 of our 751 patients (31.0 percent), and 123/751 (16.4 percent) also had hypertension, despite an initial screening out of the more severely hypertensive individuals. These figures seem fairly typical of younger post-coronary patients.10,11

However, the overall recurrence rate, combining data for high and low intensity exercise, has been some 3.6/100 person years rather than the anticipated control value of 5.75/100 person years. Our overall data have to date shown little difference between high and low intensity exercise (table 3), yet a recurrence rate as low as 3.6/100 could hardly have arisen by chance. There are three possible explanations: (1) we were dealing initially with a low risk population, (2) the dropout process has subsequently eliminated from our sample those with poor health habits, or (3) both high and low intensity exercise groups benefited from contact with the rehabilitation centers.

Critical Events

The choice of critical events has in general worked well. Where a patient has died, we have attempted to obtain a postmortem report on the cause of death, volunteers being encouraged to sign a release form for this purpose on entry to the study. In the event of sudden death, this was considered an endpoint for the subject even if the postmortem did not show a typical reinfarction. However, if cardiac arrest was followed by successful resuscitation (without residual myocardial damage), the subject was retained as an active member of the research sample. To date, there have been 14 cardiac fatalities, a rate of 0.9/100 person years, with 1 further death attributed to a noncardiac cause. In a second series of patients, many of whom were older, Kavanagh and I[12] concluded that 11 of 35 deaths had a noncardiac basis. In this latter series there were some cases that required careful exploration. For example, two vehicle accidents could have been precipitated by recurrent coronary attacks, but we were fortunately able to ascertain that in one instance our subject was a passenger, and in the other episode the subject was not held responsible for the accident.

The criteria of nonfatal recurrence were the same as for admission, and there were few problems of interpretation. A "dropout" from the high intensity group was defined as a person who:

(1) Failed to attend a single supervised exercise session over a 4-week period, despite weekly reminders;

(2) Performed less than two sessions of prescribed exercise per week;

(3) Attended less than 15 class sessions in a year;

(4) Requested withdrawal from the study.

In the low intensity exercise group, the corresponding criteria were:

(1) Gross physical activity, whether obvious or detected in weekly diaries;

(2) Absence from class sessions for more than 6 weeks despite weekly reminders;

(3) Attendance at less than 10 sessions in a year;

(4) Requested withdrawal from the study.

Practical experience showed it was necessary to recognize a further category of temporary withdrawal from the study due to such factors as:

● Medical problems (dysrhythmias, musculoskeletal problems, reevaluation);

● Vacation or temporary work more than 30 miles from a center;

● Temporary domestic problems, such as child care;

● Temporary problems due to shift work.

It was decided that each temporary withdrawal be assessed on its merits by the local center's coordinator. Except when medically contraindicated, subjects granted temporary withdrawal status were encouraged to maintain a program on their own, monitored by an exercise log, until it was practical for them to rejoin the standard program. Temporary withdrawals were typically for 2 to 6 months. If it appeared likely that a problem would persist for longer, the subject was classed as a dropout.

In the event that surgery was undertaken, subjects were again excluded from further consideration. This may have introduced some bias, in that subjects undertaking high intensity exercise were more likely to develop symptoms and thus to be referred for surgery.

Preliminary data on the status of trial participants after an average of 20 months of observation are summarized in Table 3. The required number of patients was duly recruited, but already the number of dropouts has exceeded our hopes.

According to popular belief, the dropout rate is highest in the first few months of observation. Some studies have thus given several preliminary months of exercise prior to the randomization of subjects.[1] However, the results of the southern Ontario trial to date do not support this view (table 4). The sample size is still

Table 4: Relationship Between Period of Observation and Dropout Rate--Preliminary Data from the Southern Ontario Multicentre Trial, Based on Results for an Average Period of 20 Months

Period in Study	Dropout Rate		Anticipated Residual Active Population	
	HIE Group % per 6 months	LIE Group % per 6 months	HIE Group (of initial 375)	LIE Group (of initial 375)
0-6 months	8.4	13.1	344	326
6-12	13.1	15.4	299	276
12-18	28.0	11.1	215	245
18-24	10.4	6.6	193	229
24-30	7.5	9.9	178	206
30-36	9.9	3.7	161	199
36-42	19.4	9.0	129	181
42-48	(30.0)*	(3.4)*	(91)*	(175)*
	Average for 4-year period		201	201

*Small sample.

HIE = high intensity exercise; LIE = low intensity exercise.

limited for the 3rd and 4th years of observation, but if attrition rates for these years are calculated as a percentage of the residual sample, losses seem at least as great as for the first 2 years of observation. Extrapolating current trends, we may be left with about 264 patients at the end of the 4th year, a dropout rate of 60 to 65 percent rather than the desired figure of 25 to 35 percent.

Oldridge[13] has analyzed reasons for defection from the study (table 5). As in many previous investigations, medical problems account for only 22 percent, almost half of these being noncardiac causes. A further 25 percent are unavoidable due to such factors as change of employment, leaving 42 percent attributable to psychosocial and 11 percent to other causes. The worst experience is with blue collar employees doing light work who are smokers and are inactive during their leisure time; 95 percent of such subjects defect within 2 years (table 6).

Table 5: Reasons for Defection From the Study, Based on an Analysis of Oldridge[13]

	%
Medical causes - noncardiac	8.8
cardiac	13.2
Total	22.0
Unavoidable	25.0
Psychosocial	42.0
Other	11.0

Table 6: Identification of the Exercise Dropout, Based on an Analysis of Oldridge[13]

	%
Standard dropout rate	45
Smokers	58
Smokers, blue collar work	69
Smokers, blue collar work, inactive leisure	80
Smokers, blue collar work, inactive leisure, light work	95

Many of the dropouts had surprisingly positive perceptions of the program. Nevertheless, relative to the compliers there was less enthusiasm for the program. It was also perceived as more fatiguing and less convenient with respect to occupation and domestic responsibilities.

There was almost a two-fold inter-center difference in the incidence of defections. We suggest that this relates partly to methods of recruitment (physician referral, 43.0 percent attrition, vs. the combing of cardiac wards, 55.3 percent attrition); other possible factors include differences in the average socioeconomic status of subjects attending the different centers, along with differences in the personality of the clinical staff and their degree of involvement in the rehabilitation process. A personal rapport between physician and subject is important to continuing interest in the rehabilitation program, and one of the major challenges has been to sustain such a rapport as the program has grown at the various centers.

The high dropout rate seen in the southern Ontario trial and in other studies[2] raises several practical questions: (1) Could the percentage of dropouts be reduced if investigators were paid only for subjects completing the study? (2) Can one draw conclusions about the value of exercise therapy when the majority of the subjects has not experienced it? (3) Even if exercise is of value, will it be possible to persuade the average postcoronary patient to adopt such treatment? Paradoxically, if the first two questions can be resolved, the resulting enthusiasm for exercise may be sufficient to ensure subsequent participation by the general population of postcoronary patients.

Compliance with Exercise Therapy

The term "dropout" is often used rather loosely, but when analyzing data it is important to distinguish between the dropout, the noncomplier, and the nonrespondent to an exercise program. In our particular experimental design, a few subjects in the high intensity exercise program may well have gone through the motions of participation in the formal classes, while lacking the enthusiasm to carry out their home prescription and thus to develop a significant training response. Others may have trained faithfully, yet their response was limited by severe or progressing disease. Conversely, some in the low intensity exercise group may have become contaminated by an undetected interest in vigorous activity. This last problem has been exacerbated by recent publicity concerning the merits of exercise for the "postcoronary" patient.

The general nature of the programs offered to the two groups of patients at the several centers was monitored periodically by a visiting team of physical educators. The high intensity group followed a program of dynamic exercise, particularly jogging. After a preliminary 8-week period of mild but increasing exercise, each participant was given a personal exercise prescription, based upon performance of a simple bicycle ergometer test.[14] A typical initial requirement was for some 30 minutes of activity at 60 percent of maximum oxygen intake, with progression to an intensity of 70 to 80 percent after 1 year, as clinical conditions permitted. Each subject exercised a minimum of four times per week.

During the first 2 years postinfarction, one or two of those sessions were supervised each week, thus allowing instructors to check performance, pulse rate, and symptoms, adjust the prescription if necessary, and check dysrhythmias by telemetry. During the remaining sessions, the subjects exercised on their own, at an intensity slightly below that of the formal class session, compliance being monitored by an exercise log.[15] At the larger centers, the supervised classes showed signs of becoming unmanageably large. It was thus decided that when 2 years of weekly supervised exercises had been completed, the subjects should graduate to a program of one supervised session every 4 weeks, progress over the intervening period being monitored by the exercise log.

The LIE group met weekly for light recreational activities, structured to keep pulse rates below 120 beat/min, interest being sustained at some centers by additional sessions devoted to relaxation techniques including hypnosis and yoga.

It was originally envisaged that all participants would have regular and detailed physiological assessment, including rebreathing assessments of cardiac output,[14] with quality control assured by regular inter-laboratory biological standardization.[16] When the study was expanded from four to seven centers, it was decided that the costs of equipping and maintaining three additional laboratories were unwarranted. Accordingly, detailed physiological information will be available for only a sub-sample of subjects. Nevertheless, all participants have carried out regular progressive bicycle ergometer tests with heart rate recording, and this provides a combined assessment of compliance and biological responsiveness. One problem in applying this standard is that an ever-increasing proportion of our subjects has been receiving beta-blocking drugs such as propranolol. Often, the referring physician has agreed to our request for a tapered withdrawal of the

drug to allow exercise testing, but in a few instances
this was not possible. The best that could then be accomplished was a comparison of performances at the same dose
of propranolol.

To date we have only analyzed physiological data for
subjects who have had simultaneous measurements of oxygen
consumption. Levels of cardiorespiratory fitness varied
considerably among subjects. Accordingly, all heart
rates were reported at a directly measured or closely
interpolated value of 1.25 l/min STPD. The average data
showed a progressive decrease of heart rate in the high
intensity exercise group. In our first analysis (table
7), this was equivalent to a 13.2 percent increase of
predicted maximum oxygen over 2 years, although a larger
series has now shown an average gain of some 23 percent.[16] Both analyses showed a suggestion of early improvement in the control group, presumably due to such
factors as continued natural healing, test habituation,
and possibly a small effect of the recreational program
on physical condition.

Table 7: Preliminary Data on Changes in Exercise Response
Over First 2 Years of Participation in Multicentre Trial

	HIE Group		LIE Group	
	f_h, 1.25 (beats/min)*	Predicted VO_2 (max) (l./min)*	f_h, 1.25 (beats/min)*	Predicted VO_2 (max) (l./min)*
Initial	119.4	2.01	119.2	2.02
1 year	115.5	2.16 (+ 7.4%)	117.2	2.09 (+3.9%)
2 years	112.6	2.27 (+13.2%)**	115.7	2.15 (+6.6%)

*Absolute values distorted by propranolol in a few subjects, but relative
change valid.

**Differs significantly from result for LIE group.

Heart rate at an interpolated oxygen consumption of 1.25 l./min STPD,
and maximum oxygen intake as predicted by Astrand nomogram.

HIE = high intensity exercise; LIE = low intensity exercise.

Thus, over the first year, the difference in behavior
of high and low intensity exercise groups was quite small.
At 2 years, the difference was larger and statistically
significant in both analyses. This emphasizes the point
that in the postcoronary patient training responses are
slow to develop. Our multicentre study data show no gains
of cardiac stroke volume until the second 6 months of
training.[17] An earlier study looked at 13 postcoronary

patients who had prepared themselves for marathon participation;[18] in some of these individuals, maximum oxygen intake continued to increase for 3 and even 4 years.

It thus seems fallacious to look for a rapid improvement of prognosis with exercise rehabilitation. We do not know the precise lag period between a gain of physical condition and any possible influence on prognosis; but, if a minimum of 1 year is needed for conditioning we should certainly exclude from our comparisons reinfarctions sustained over a shorter period. It seems significant that in a previous evaluation of exercise rehabilitation, Kavanagh et al.[19] noted a reinfarction rate of 3.11 percent for the first year of observation, 2.58 percent for the second year, 1.50 percent for the third to the fifth years, and only 0.81 percent for the sixth to eighth years of exercise.

Activity Status of Patients Suffering Reinfarction

Noting these comments on compliance and response, when did the reinfarctions occur in the southern Ontario trial? Our preliminary results show that a number developed within a few weeks of recruitment, and 20 of the first 50 events were seen within 12 months of recruitment (table 8). In my view, none of these patients had trained long enough to realize the possible benefits of exercise.

Theoretically, all of the remaining 30 recurrences occurred in patients who were still exercising. However, in practice, many were dropouts. While the effects of training can be dissipated by a few weeks of inactivity, it takes a minimum of 8 weeks (longer if a temporary withdrawal) to probe a patient's excuses and realize that he has dropped out of the project. In fact, 16 of the remaining 30 infarcts were in patients who had made almost no attempt to attend classes over the previous 3 months. If we exclude recruits with less than 1 year's experience of exercise and those with poor recent compliance, we are currently left with only 14 critical events, 10 in the high intensity and 4 in the low intensity exercise group. Repeated laboratory exercise data were available for 10 of these 14 subjects (table 9). An improvement of physical condition was seen in five of the six high intensity exercisers, but there was also a significant decrease in exercise heart rate in two of the four low intensity exercisers.

This chapter has considered only results for an average of 20 months of participation, and numbers should be

Table 8: Compliance and Duration of Exercise in Those Patients Sustaining a Reinfarction--Preliminary Data from Southern Ontario Multicentre Trial for an Average of 20 Months

Event	Exercise Status		HIE Group		LIE Group	
			Events	Compliance* %	Events	Compliance* %
Fatal reinfarction	Active	>12/12	1	100	0	-
		<12/12	2	78	4	78
	Inactive		3	8	2	0
Nonfatal recurrence	Active	>12/12	9	76	4	83
		<12/12	9	85	5	76
	Inactive		6	16	5	6
Total recurrences	Active	>12/12	10	78	4	83
		<12/12	11	84	9	77
	Inactive		9	13	7	4

*Based on reported attendance for 3 months preceding event.

Average period of observation = 20 months.

HIE = high intensity exercise; LIE = low intensity exercise.

Table 9: Changes in Interpolated Heart Rate at an Oxygen Consumption of 1.25/min STPD. Patients Participating in Experiment for Longer than 12 Months

HIE Group		LIE Group	
Initial	Final	Initial	Final
127/min	115/min	110/min	103/min
decrease in 5/6		decrease in 2/4	

HIE = high intensity exercise; LIE = low intensity exercise.

284

approximately doubled when all patients have been followed for 4 years.* Nevertheless, despite recruitment of the stipulated 740 patients, we will obviously fall far short of the comparison required for our original statistical proof--56 valid incidents in the low intensity exercise group, and 28 valid incidents in the high intensity exercise group. To be certain of observing this many events in subjects recruited for at least 1 year, complying with the program, and showing a physiological response, a population of at least 4,500 would be needed.

Even a study of this order might leave unanswered the possibility that exercise is beneficial for some classes of infarct and not for others. Although numbers are still small, our data suggest that vigorous activity has an adverse effect upon the chances of a fatal recurrence in patients with more than 0.2 mV ST segmental depression during exercise[20], and the magnitude of this effect is sufficient to obscure any favorable influence of physical activity upon patients with less severe coronary disease.

Lastly, we must ask whether we (and other investigators) have chosen the most appropriate critical events. Death and reinfarction are easy to measure, but the average patient is concerned more with the quality than with the quantity of his remaining years. We suspect that exercise has improved the quality of life for many of our patients[21] but as yet have no strong documentation of this belief.

Future Options

What lessons for future planning can be drawn from the southern Ontario experience? Certainly, our study is yielding a wealth of information on the practical problems of study organization and design. Pessimists might conclude that a controlled study to determine the influence of exercise upon the rate of reinfarction is logistically impossible, accepting in its place the evidence of a low reinfarction rate in uncontrolled exercise trials.[19] Optimists might attempt to meet the requirements of large numbers by pooling data from various current controlled studies, ignoring obvious differences of philosophy and protocol. But from a scientific point of view, the only satisfactory course is to regard existing experiments as pilot trials, using the data obtained to design an effective and statistically conclusive study.

*Since it appears impossible for the study to answer the problem posed, the final cohort of subjects may be followed for 3 rather than 4 years.

In view of the number of patients required and the associated high costs, such an investigation would have to be tackled on an international basis. Hopefully, our discussions may set the stage for such an undertaking.

References

1. Naughton J: The national exercise and heart disease project. Manual of Operations. Washington, DC, George Washington University, 1978

2. Wilhelmsen L, Sanne H, Elmfeldt D, Grimby G, Tibblin G, Wadel H: A controlled trial of physical training after myocardial infarction. Prev Med 4, 491-508, 1975

3. Kentala E: Physical fitness and feasibility of physical rehabilitation after myocardial infarction in men of working age. Ann Clin Res 4, (suppl 9), 1-84, 1972

4. Rechnitzer PA, Sangal SA, Cunningham DA, Andrew G, Buck C, Jones N, Kavanagh T, Parker J, Shephard RJ, Yuhasz MS: A controlled prospective study of the effect of endurance training on the recurrence rate of myocardial infarction--a description of experimental design. Am J Epidemiol 102, 358-365, 1975

5. Rechnitzer PA, Pickard HA, Pavio A, Yuhasz MS, Cunningham DA: Long term followup of survival and recurrence rates following myocardial infarction in exercising and control subjects. Circulation 45, 853-857, 1972

6. Wald A: Sequential Analysis. New York, John Wiley, 1947

7. Norris RM, Caughey DE, Deeming LW, Mercer CJ, Scott PJ: Coronary prognostic index for predicting survival after recovery from acute myocardial infarction. Lancet (ii), 485-487, 1970

8. Williamson JS, Bauman DJ, Tsagaris TJ: A comparison of hemodynamic and angiographic indices of left ventricular performance in patients with coronary artery disease. Cardiology 63, 220-236, 1978

9. Berman DS, Amsterdam EA, Mason DT: Detection of myocardial ischemia by rest and exercise. Thallium 201 scintigraphy. In, Exercise in Cardiovascular Health and Disease (Amsterdam EA, Wilmore JH, deMaria AN, eds). New York, Yorke Books, 1977

10. Weinblatt E, Shapiro S, Frank CW, Sager RV: Prognosis of men after first myocardial infarction: mortality and recurrence in relation to selected parameters. Am J Public Health 58, 1329-1347, 1968

11. Stamler JS: Clofibrate and niacin in coronary heart disease. (For Coronary Drug Project.) JAMA 231, 360-373, 1975

12. Kavanagh T, Shephard RJ, Chisholm AW, Qureshi S, Kennedy J: Prognostic indices for ischemic heart disease in patients enrolled in an exercise-centered rehabilitation program. Am J Cardiol 44, 1230-1240, 1979

13. Oldridge N: The problem of compliance. Med Sci Sports (in press, 1979)

14. Jones NL, Campbell EJM, Robertson DG, Edwards RHT: Clinical Exercise Testing. Philadelphia, W.B. Saunders, 1975

15. Shephard RJ: Alive, Man! The Physiology of Physical Activity. Springfield, C.C. Thomas, 1972

16. Cunningham DA, Ingram KJ, Rechnitzer PA, Jones NL, Shephard RJ, Sangal S, Andrew G, Buck C, Kavanagh T, Parker JO, Yuhasz MS: Effects of a 2-year program of exercise training on cardiovascular fitness and recurrence rates in post-myocardial infarction patients. An interim report. Cardiologia 62, 136-137, 1977

17. Paterson D, Shephard RJ, Cunningham D, Jones N, Andrew G: Effects of mild and vigorous physical training upon cardiovascular function following infarction. J Appl Physiol 47, 482-489, 1979

18. Kavanagh T, Shephard RJ, Kennedy J: Characteristics of post-coronary marathon runners. Ann NY Acad Sci 301, 455-465, 1977

19. Kavanagh T, Shephard RJ, Kennedy J, Qureshi S: Are the benefits of exercise in post-coronary rehabilitation an artefact of patient selection? Cardiologia 62, 84-85, 1977

20. Shephard RJ: Recurrence of myocardial infarction in an exercising population. Br Heart J 42, 133-138, 1979

21. Kavanagh T, Shephard RJ, Tuck J, Qureshi S: Depression following myocardial infarction--the effects of distance running. Ann NY Acad Sci 301, 1029-1038, 1977

21
ENDPOINT CONSIDERATIONS

Albert Oberman, M.D.

Discussion of endpoints forces us into the realities of a clinical trial in terms of the feasibility of newer diagnostic techniques and necessary commitments both in effort and in costs. I will review possible cardiovascular and scoioeconomic endpoints in relative order of importance and comment on the salient features of each endpoint. Because of the complexities in assessing clinical trials relating physical conditioning to rehabilitation, one must be assured that training effects have taken place. In a prescribed exercise program, endpoints must be predicated on the achievement of a certain degree of fitness. Therefore, major variables relating to physical training must be carefully documented as well.

Cardiovascular Endpoints

Mortality

Without doubt, mortality provides <u>the</u> answer. Some critics would opt for total mortality while others insist on subdivision into cardiovascular (ICDA code #390-458) and noncardiovascular deaths. Cardiovascular death could be attributed to heart disease (ICDA code #390-398, 402, 404, and 410-429). All medical records pertaining to the cause of death should be available for review by an impartial panel of experts. Cardiovascular deaths should be classified as sudden or nonsudden on the basis of the duration of the terminal episode and prior health status of the patient. An abundance of definitions exists for sudden death, but the usual categories include instantaneous, within 1 hour, within 3 hours or within 24 hours.[1]

Of further interest would be the occurrence of cardiac
arrest within the context of the study. Without resuscitation efforts, primary cardiac arrest generally is
equated to sudden death.[2] With our current procedures
for completion of death certificates, further breakdown
of causes of death would not prove meaningful. Obviously, the use of mortality endpoints as opposed to a change
in some quantitative measure assessed at baseline will
greatly escalate sample size requirements. This issue
will be addressed later by Dr. Hyde in discussing sample
size considerations.

Morbidity

Hospitalizations. In terms of rehabilitation, the
need for hospitalization and related costs provide
essential information by which physical conditioning
programs can be judged. Variables such as number of
hospitalizations, length of hospitalizations, expenses
incurred, and subsequent disability days constitute
appropriate indices of morbidity. Surgical treatment by
coronary artery bypass grafting procedures would be of
special interest from the standpoint of rehabilitation
as well as medical therapeutic failure.

Myocardial infarction. Though based on "softer" data,
myocardial infarction can certainly be measured objectively and provide a satisfactory endpoint for analysis.
A recent expert committee on clinical nomenclature[2]
based guidelines for the diagnosis on history, ECG, and
enzymes as noted in table 1. Definite acute myocardial

Table 1: Guidelines for the Diagnosis of Myocardial
Infarction

	Unequivocal	Equivocal
ECG	(a) Persistent Q, QS waves (b) Evolving injury current lasting longer than 1 day	(a) Stationary injury current (b) Transient Q waves (c) Symmetrical T wave inversion (d) Conduction disturbance
Enzymes	(a) Serial rise and fall properly related to specific enzymes (b) Elevation cardiospecific isoenzymes	Elevation initially without subsequent fall
History	Typical or atypical	

infarction is considered present when unequivocal ECG
changes and/or unequivocal enzyme changes supplemented

by either typical or atypical history occur. Possible infarction is diagnosed when equivocal ECG changes persist more than 24 hours with or without equivocal enzyme changes but with a compatible history.

Left ventricular function. Left ventricular dysfunction can certainly be defined clinically by the following variables, either separately or in some combination: tachycardia, third heart sound, dyspnea on exertion, paroxysmal nocturnal dyspnea, orthopnea, edema, and cardiomegaly on the plain chest film. The simplest measure would be calculation of heart volume by chest X-ray. This has been related both to left ventricular function and prognosis.[3,4] Indirect measures of left ventricular function include the total time on the treadmill and an inappropriate increment in systolic blood pressure. The PEP:LVET ratio or other parameters measured from the systolic time intervals may be of value but have not gained wide acceptance.[5]

Another published technique is the measurement of cardiac output by a carbon dioxide rebreathing method providing measurements of cardiac output both at rest and during exercise.[6] This technique requires further validation in coronary patients. This method involves measurement of carbon dioxide production from the volume and concentration in the expired air by a rapid single breath gas analysis and carbon dioxide content. The rebreathing procedure is used to obtain mixed venous PCO_2. However, the requirement for further validation in coronary patients as well as the complexity and costs of the routine may override the ability to gain valuable information noninvasively.

Using noninvasive procedures, it is now possible to refine and quantify left ventricular dysfunction. The M-mode echocardiogram provides information on left ventricular status; various studies have correlated the volume of the left ventricle with that found at cardiac catheterization. This approximation works out fairly well, by assuming an ellipsoid shape and cubing the end diastolic and end systolic diameters or using a regression formula to obtain the ejection fraction (stroke volume/ end diastolic volumes). More specific hemodynamic measurements can be made, but involve a number of assumptions. The prediction can be inaccurate because of sampling an area contracting excessively to compensate for distal hypodyskinesia or, conversely, because of a poorly contracting area.

The more sophisticated technique, two dimensional echocardiography, is more expensive, provides lower resolution, and is still in a developmental state for general usage. Even the two dimensional echocardiogram is difficult to complete in patients with chronic obstructive lung disease because of the air barrier to sound waves or in patients with chest deformities. The complexities and problems with reliability of current techniques result in missing data on a substantial segment of the population and negate the value of echocardiography for exercise trials in the immediate future. Angiography (table 2) offers the most direct approach for left ventricular assessment-ejection fraction, stroke output, pressures and volumes, and regional contractility--but necessitates an invasive, costly procedure with associated radiation hazards. Angiography may be a needless repetition for those patients who underwent this diagnostic procedure as part of their workup at the time of myocardial infarction. There are inherent errors associated with this procedure such as the influence of the injection medium; however, it offers the important

Table 2:   Endpoint Data Available from Angiography

Endpoint Variables

LV pressures
LV volume
LV ejection fraction
Stroke output
Mitral regurgitation
Contractibility
   gross
   regional
Coronary lesions
Collateral circulation

---

advantage of direct visualization of the coronary arteries and collateral circulation. From the standpoint of study design, the ability to preclude later "crossover" to coronary artery surgery, a confusing feature of such trials, by this initial assessment could prove very worthwhile. For example, patients with substantial left main coronary artery lesions could be identified immediately, decreasing the future likelihood of coronary artery surgery during the clinical trial evaluation.

The most recent addition to the cardiovascular diagnostic armamentarium, the radionuclide scanning technique, offers an invaluable tool for developing endpoints. Using the gated blood pool method, one can inject technetium-labeled red blood cells or albumin and

identify systolic and disatolic volumes over time, obtain
regional wall motion in selected segments, and calculate
the ejection fraction. All variables can be quantified
and lend themselves to multivariate analyses. The technique is noninvasive, without anatomical limitations,
permits multiple serial studies, and appears to be without significant radiation hazard. The frequency and
severity of angina does not always correlate with the
extent of disease or left ventricular performance.
Therefore, the ability of the myocardium to contract and
increase the ejection fraction with exercise provides
critical functional information which is valid, reproducible, and quantifiable, relating directly to functional
capacity and the goals of rehabilitation. This technique
seems uniquely suitable for a serial evaluation of exercise treatment.

The simpler thallium technique with exercise enables
one to identify scars and reversible ischemic areas in
terms of percent of total areas involved. This can be
relayed directly onto a computer tape for calculation.
The expense and logistics of this routine at present preclude its implementation at a number of centers without
active research facilities. One would expect these techniques to develop rapidly in the immediate future, providing information not previously obtainable.

Angina. Angina (table 3) can be classified in terms
of severity (frequency, amount of nitroglycerin required
per week, functional class, treadmill state); instability

Table 3: Classification of Angina

Severity

Frequency
No. nitroglycerin tablets/week
Workload to induce

Unstable

Nocturnal
At rest
Prolonged

Intractable

(nocturnal, at rest, lasting 15 minutes or more); or
intractable (nonresponsive to optimal medical therapy).
Ischemia can be assessed by ECG signs with exercise such
as ST depression, chest pain, or even perhaps R wave in-
crements[7] either separately or combined with relative
workload. The heart rate systolic blood pressure product
approximates myocardial oxygen consumption and provides
a valuable index for anginal threshold. Repetitive thallium radionuclide scans identify underperfused ischemic
areas induced by exercise and relieved by rest and offer
a possibility for endpoint definition in the near future.

Atherosclerotic lesions

At the present time the atherosclerotic lesion can
only be identified appropriately by coronary arteriography, although calcification can be qualitatively defined with fluoroscopy and even on a plain chest film
with proper equipment.[8,9] Coronary calcification detected noninvasively can be used in conjunction with
exercise testing for improving the predictive accuracy
of arteriographic findings.[8] Two-dimensional echocardiography also holds promise for identifying lesions in
selected locations. In the distant future, positron
imaging with automated tomography, using a cyclotron or
other techniques not yet developed, may open new vistas.
Meanwhile, the atherosclerotic lesions can be quantified
using various techniques such as that developed by Brown
and coworkers[11] at the University of Washington for segmental artery analysis to evaluate various therapeutic
interventions in coronary disease.

Lesions are traced from two perpendicular projections
using 35 mm cineangiographic views and transmitted to the
computer adjusting for magnification by using the catheter diameter. Views are modified creating spatial repre-
sentation of the vessel. Assuming an elliptical lumen,
the absolute and percent reduction of diameter or cross-
sectional areas of stenosis can be computed (figure 1).
More complex functions such as the integrated atheroma-
tous mass, resistance, and orifice resistance area can
also be calculated. It should be realized that errors
of overlapping vessels and other technical difficulties
limit these measurements to 60 to 90 percent of available
arteriograms if one is willing to accept a single projection in some patients.

Workers at the University of Alabama Medical Center[12]
have used a simpler technique employing a vernier caliper
also correcting for magnification by the size of the
catheter in the ostium. The degree of stenosis can be
calculated by a formula which has been validated in postmortem studies. There are innumerable ways of assessing
the vasculature on the angiogram and collateral circulation, such as number of vessels of certain size, density

294

	Proximal	Distal	Minimum	Sten	Atheroma		
LAO (MM)	3.268	2.649	0.845	71.4%	Length	=	13.578 MM
RAO (MM)	3.015	2.888	0.751	74.6%	Mass	=	45.6274 MM^3
AREA (MM^2)	7.739	6.009	0.503	92.7%	Mass/Length	=	3.3604

Resistance (MMHG/CC/SEC) = 6.5991   (Poiseuille)
Resistance/Length = 4.8602   Resistance Ratio = 29.4728

Flow (CC/SEC)	Orifice Res.	Total Pressure Drop (MMHG)
1	14.7471	21.3462
2	29.4941	72.1865
3	44.2412	152.5210

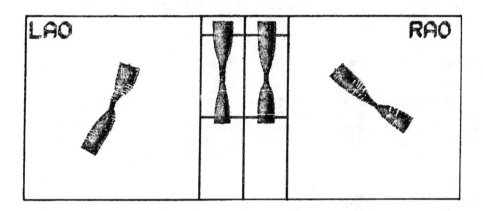

Figure 1: Example of the hard copy printout of segmental
analysis of coronary artery lesion. The lesions are portrayed to scale in the outer boxes, with a scale dimension
of 3 cm along the box edge. The inner panels show matched
portions of the two views stretched out to true length
at the same scale. The computations are explained in the
text.

of vessels, and so forth.[13] The collaterals provide a
critical perspective suggested in the experimental literature which has eluded investigators. With better equipment, refined methods, and the possibility of obtaining
films during exercise, measurement of collateral circulation would be of inestimable value. The promotion of
collateral circulation through exercise training has long
been thought to be an important but poorly documented
protective mechanism for patients with coronary disease.

Dysrhythmias

Because of their frequency in exercise sessions and
presumed importance as a prognostic factor, dysrhythmias,
primarily premature ventricular beats, deserve consideration as independent endpoints. Measurement should include evaluation at rest, during exercise (exercise test),
and throughout the day (24-hour Holter monitoring).
These methods permit assessment of frequency, focus,
coupling interval, and patterns in different situations
throughout daily activities.

Socioeconomic Factors

Assessment of rehabilitation cannot be complete without attention to non-medical indices of success (table
4). The most objective and simplest measures are employment status including occupation, hours worked per week,

Table 4: Socioeconomic Endpoints for Rehabilitation

Employment Status

   Occupation
   Hours worked
   Relative work capacity

Income Distribution

Social Activities

Psychologic Attributes

   Attitude toward life and illness
   Anxiety, depression
   Personality traits

---

and ability to perform on the job. These measures of work should be considered not only absolutely, but relative to the patient's physical capacity so that one can determine whether he has been rehabilitated to the fullest extent possible. Occupations including housekeeping and other duties performed predominantly by women must be considered.

Income and its distribution by family members are important socioeconomic indices. It is entirely possible for the income to remain approximately the same but now derived from a working mother or sources of disability compensation, greatly influencing a patient's lifestyle. Scales of attitude toward life and illness and social activities determining the quality of one's life must be ascertained. Certain personality characteristics reflected by anxiety, depression, hypochondriasis, and Type A-B trials should also be included since these are frequently related to rehabilitation success. Not infrequently, the psychological rather than the physiological variables are the limiting factors in daily activities.

Training Effects

Invariably the question arises of the relationship of exercise training to endpoints. Were the endpoints associated with the magnitude of the training effect? Were insignificant differences attributable to lack of training or dropouts? A clinical trial on coronary disease dealing with the effects of a prescribed exercise program on rehabilitation by definition concerns fitness. Training responses must be evaluated as necessary intermediates to accomplish the proposed endpoints. In addition to maximal work capacity, cardiovascular fitness can be measured by heart rate, blood pressure, and myocardial energy requirements at rest and at various exercise levels. Attendance records for the training program and heart rate targets provide important ancillary information. In addition, careful records must be kept on drug usage, especially those commonly used agents, such as propranolol, which can modify both fitness measures and endpoints. Provisions must be made to take into account these factors when determining study outcomes.

Summary

Table 5 displays a possible array of endpoints derived from a number of diagnostic procedures, some relatively new and unexplored from the standpoint of clinical trials. The design, magnitude, and value of any clinical trial of exercise for coronary patients depend on the appropriate selection of these endpoints.

Table 5: Diagnostic Procedures Required for Acquisition of Endpoints

Endpoints	Question-naires	Physical Exam	ECG	Chest Film	Multi-Stage Exercise Test	Syst. Time Interv.	Echo	Angio-Graphy	Radio-Nuclide Scanning Test
Mortality	X								
Morbidity									
Myocardial infarction	X		X					X	X
Left vent. function	X	X		X	X	X	X	X	X
Angina-Ischemia	X				X				X
Ath lesion-vasculature				X				X	
Dysrhythmia			X		X				
Socioeconomic									
Occupation	X								
Income	X								
Social activity	X								
Psychologic	X								
Fitness	X		X		X				

References

1. Prineas RJ, Blackburn H (eds): Sudden Coronary Death Outside Hospital. American Heart Association Monograph, no 47, 1975

2. Joint International Society and Federation of Cardiology/World Health Organization Task Force on Standardization of Clinical Nomenclature: Nomenclature and criteria for diagnosis of ischemic heart disease. Circulation 59:607-609, 1979

3. Oberman A: The natural history of coronary disease. In, Coronary Artery Disease: Recognition and Management (Rackley CE, Russell RO Jr, eds). New York, Futura Publ Co, 1979, p 1

4. Hammermeister KE, Chikos PM, Fisher L, Dodge HT: Relationship of cardiothoracic ration and plain film heart volume to late survival. Circulation 59(1): 89-95, 1979

5. Lewis RP, Rutgers SE, Forester WF, Boudoulas H: A critical review of the systolic time intervals. Circulation 56:146-158, 1977

6. Franciosa JA, Ragan DO, Rubestone SJ: Validation of the CO_2 rebreathing method for measuring cardiac output in patients with hypertension or heart failure. J Lab Clin Med 672-682, October, 1976

7. Bonoris PE, Greenberg PS, Castellancet MD, Ellestad MH: Significance of changes in R wave amplitude during treadmill stress testing: angiographic correlation. Am J Cardiol 41:846, 1978

8. Aldrich RF, Brensike JF, Battaglini JW, et al: Coronary calcifications in the detection of coronary artery disease and comparison with electrocardiographic exercise testing: results from the National Heart, Lung, and Blood Institute's type II coronary intervention study. Circulation 59:1113-1124, 1979

9. Souza AS, Bream PR, Elliott LP: Chest film detection of coronary artery calcification (CAC): the value of the CAC triangle. Radiology 129:7-10, 1978

10. Brown BG, Bolson E, Frimer M, Dodge HT: Quantitative coronary arteriography: estimation of dimensions, hemodynamic resistance, and atheroma mass of coronary artery lesions using the arteriogram and digital computation. Circulation 55:329-337, 1977

11. Rafflenbeul W, Smith LR, Rogers WJ, Mantle JA, Rackley CE, Russell RO Jr: Quantitative coronary arteriography: coronary anatomy of patients with unstable angina pectoris reexamined 1 year after optimal medical therapy. Am J Cardiol 43:699-707, 1979

12. Maurer BJ, Oberman A, Jones WB, Kouchoukos NT, Reeves TJ: Clinical and angiographic followup of patients with saphenous vein bypass graft. Circulation 48 (suppl IV), 1973

22

SAMPLE SIZE CONSIDERATIONS

John Hyde III, Ph.D.

The process of determining a sample size for a study is usually an iterative procedure. An initial estimate is proposed, the design is evaluated and modified, and revised sample size estimates are derived. The planning of a major study can involve a number of cycles.

The final outcome of the deliberations will depend on factors such as the relative importance of competing objectives and the practical limitations of money, energy, and technology. Because of these unquantifiables, I cannot hope to come up with a single specific proposal on how large a prospective study of rehabilitation needs to be.

I will instead take on two objectives. In the design stage of a study it is useful to know what aspects of design influence the sample size and to know the sensitivity of the sample size to each of these influences. So I will first review the sample size "recipe" with an eye toward quantifying the way each ingredient affects the outcome. Second, I will consider a few major endpoints and present some broad ranges of the number of patients likely to be required for each endpoint.

Factors Affecting Sample Size

For a given endpoint, the sample size determination requires the investigators to specify how clearly they wish to discern differences between the responses of the treatment and control groups. It is also necessary to have information about the properties of the endpoint itself and to know what can be expected of the population to be studied. Let me review these items in detail.

First, there is the Type I error rate, often referred to as alpha. This can be thought of as the false positive rate; the probability that one will decide, erroneously, that the treatment and control groups differ, when in fact they are not really different. The investigators specify what the error rate should be. This choice may be guided by custom, by the editorial policy of one's favorite journal, or by the skepticism of the intended audience. If this error rate is kept small, one can argue more convincingly that any observed difference is not simply a random fluctuation. Current convention says that this rate should not exceed 5 percent, and preferably it should be lower.

The other side of the coin is the Type II error rate, often called beta, which can be thought of as the false negative rate. The quantity one minus beta is referred to as the power. Suppose that one fails to find an expected treatment effect. How confident can one be that the effect of treatment actually is less than that which was expected? The answer depends on the false negative rate. If the rate is high, then a negative result is likely in any event, so it cannot be viewed as particularly strong evidence against the existence of the expected treatment effect. Ideally, an experiment should provide useful information no matter what the outcome. The application of this principle points to using low values for both error rates. A 5 percent error rate (a power of 95 percent) is a desirable objective.

Figure 1 indicates how the sample size depends on the error rates for a hypothetical experiment. It is apparent that as one gets closer to zero error rates, one pays increasingly steeper premiums for improvements in the error rates. For example, lowering the alpha error from 5 percent to 2 percent increases the sample size by 21 percent, while the penultimate percent alone costs an additional 16 percent. One can also see how the sample size can be reduced by sacrificing power. Compared to a study with 95 percent power, the size needed for 90 percent power is 19 percent less; for 85 percent power it is 31 percent less; and for 80 percent power it is 39 percent less.

The anticipated difference between treatment and control values is crucial in determining the needed study size. It turns out that the sample size is quite sensitive to this difference; it is approximately inversely proportional to the square of the difference. In order to improve the sensitivity of a study so that it can detect treatment effects which are half as large, the

302

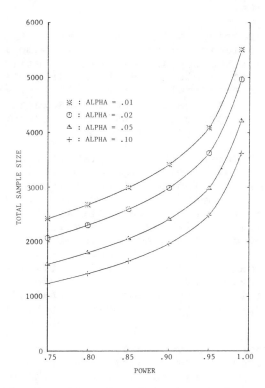

Figure 1: Total sample size versus power for different values of alpha. Twenty percent control rate with 25 percent reduction.

sample size needs to be roughly quadrupled. Alternatively, small percentage changes in the anticipated treatment effect necessitate twice the percentage change in the sample size. This magnifying effect is sometimes called the delta-squared phenomenon.

It is important to note that the anticipated treatment effect should incorporate the degradation in response to treatment due to non-adherence. Thus, if one-third of the subjects in the treatment group do not adhere to therapy, the anticipated treatment effect should be taken to be only two thirds of the effect expected from complete adherence. (A more precise analysis would modify this value based on the rate at which patients go off therapy and on the time it takes for the treatment to reach full effect. In planning an actual study these refinements should be taken into account, but they are less important for the present general discussion.) This approach assumes an analysis which does not exclude non-adherers. Unless there is overwhelming evidence that non-adherers should have had the same response as adherers if they

303

had not dropped out, the preferred analysis includes all randomized patients.

I have been referring to the "anticipated" treatment effect in the calculation of sample size. Sometimes a smaller effect than the one anticipated may still be of keen interest if its existence can be clearly established. In such situations this smaller treatment effect should be used in the calculations instead of the anticipated one. It should be kept in mind that the increased sensitivity will require a larger sample size.

The sample size depends on the variability of the endpoint being evaluated. The estimation of variability is frequently a major contributor to uncertainty about the sample size needed to provide the specified statistical properties. Here it is useful to distinguish between binary and non-binary variables. Binary variables, which can take on one of only two possible values, are exemplified by mortality. The mean of a binary variable is simply a proportion or a rate. The variability of a binary variable is determined by this rate. For studies looking for a fractional reduction in the rate, the sample size is approximately inversely proportional to the rate.

On the other hand, the variability of a non-binary variable is measured by its standard deviation. The sample size is proportional to the square of the standard deviation. It is important that the standard deviation be relevant for the way the endpoint will be used. If one is looking for changes in exercise performance, then the standard deviation should be measured for change in exercise test performance, not the (smaller) standard deviation for a single exercise test. If groups are being compared, the standard deviation should be for a similar population, not for an individual or for a more homogeneous or heterogeneous population. The standard deviation should not be confused with the standard error.

It is convenient to graph the sample size against the ratio of treatment effect to standard deviation, the delta/sigma ratio (figure 2). A ratio of one corresponds to the mean of one group, being at about the 85th percentile of the other. If the ratio is 0.5, the mean of one group is at the 70th percentile of the other. If the ratio is 0.25, one group's mean is at the 60th percentile of the other.

Finally, there are unavoidable losses of various sorts. Certain measurements may not be obtained at the right time, and patients may simply vanish. With good organization and aggressive followup, losses of this kind should be minor.

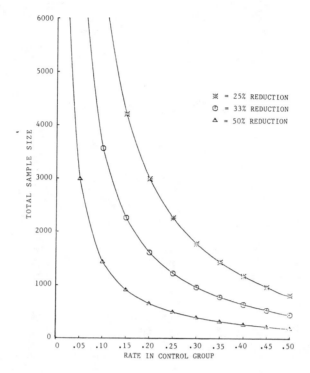

Figure 2: Total sample size for a non-binary variable versus delta/sigma. Both error rates set at 0.05.

Sample Sizes for Selected Endpoints

Now let us look at these issues in the context of cardiovascular rehabilitation. Consider the endpoint death. Figure 3 shows some sample sizes needed for a test with both error rates set at 5 percent. The horizontal axis gives the death rate in the control group. Three curves are shown corresponding to treatments which reduce the death rate by 25 percent, 33 percent or 50 percent of the control rate.

Suppose we are planning a trial in which we expect the death rate to be 0.10 in the control group and where we expect the treatment to reduce mortality by 50 percent, but with only two-thirds adhering, so that the expected death rate in the treatment group is 0.067. To obtain 5 percent error rates, a sample of around 3,600 is indicated. Note the sensitivity to the treatment effect: should we wish to have the same sensitivity to an effective 25 percent mortality reduction (50 percent ideal reduction with 50 percent adherence, or 33 percent ideal reduction with 75 percent adherence) almost twice as

305

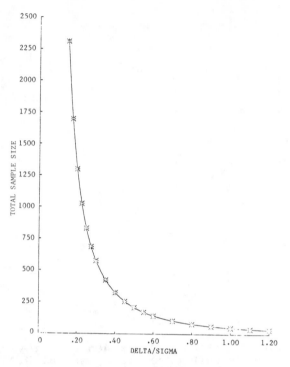

Figure 3: Total sample size versus control rate for three different treatment effects. Both error rates set at 0.05.

large a study is called for. Also, consider what might happen if overall mortality turns out to be lower than expected, so that the control group has a death rate of only 0.07. Then the original 3,600 turns out to be only 60 percent of the required size. However, a doubling of the control rate cuts the sample size by about half.

Next consider the endpoint of return to work. With the charts given here, it is more convenient to talk about the fraction which does not return to work. Some studies have shown that one might expect 20 percent of the control patients not to return to work and that rehabilitation might reduce this rate by a third. Thus the situation is very similar to that for studying mortality, and adherence of 75 percent points to a sample size of around 3,000. However, there is evidence that those in strenuous or lower class jobs may show a higher fraction not returning to work, say 40 percent, and that exercise could cut this in half. The higher control rate means that perhaps 650 patients may suffice to show a benefit of treatment if adherence is 67 percent, and 1,200 would be needed if adherence is 50 percent.

306

For maximal work during bicycle exercise, we might expect the difference between treatment and control groups to be 10 percent of the initial work output. It appears to be reasonable to take the standard deviation for change to be about 15 percent. This implies that the delta/sigma ratio is around 0.67, so that about 100 patients are called for. Should it be desired to have the same sensitivity to a difference of 7 percent or if the standard deviation is 20 percent, about 200 patients would be needed.

For submaximal heart rate we might expect the treatment group to decrease by an additional 3 percent to 5 percent over the control group. Variability may range from 5 percent to 10 percent. Therefore, indicated sample sizes range from 75 to 600 with an average size of around 200.

Other endpoints could be studied similarly, the only limitation for planning being the availability of good estimates of treatment effects and variability.

Summary

1. The sample size is very sensitive to the effect one wishes to detect, to the variability of the endpoint, and to adherence. These factors should be determined carefully in order to make the most meaningful sample size calculations. The sample size for a binary variable depends strongly on the frequency of the event, so that the selection of the patient population, the length of the study, and the exact definition of the endpoint should all be chosen with their impact on sample size clearly in mind.

2. To detect an effective 33 percent decline in mortality when the control rate is 0.10, 3,600 patients are needed. An effective mortality reduction of 25 percent (e.g., 50 percent ideal reduction subject to 50 percent adherence) would require about twice as large a study. The sample size is nearly inversely proportional to the control rate.

3. The situation for detecting changes in the fraction not returning to work is similar to the situation for mortality. However, studying patients in strenuous or lower class jobs may permit substantial reductions in the needed numbers.

4. Non-binary endpoints can get by with much smaller sample sizes than can the binary variables above. For a difference of 5 percent in heart rate change,

around 200 patients are indicated, but the number can range from 75 to 600 depending on the particular situation. For a 10 percent difference in work output change, 100 to 200 patients may suffice.

5. Using a lower power of 85 percent (a 15 percent false negative rate) would reduce the sample size by 30 percent, but at the expense of increasing the chances of missing a real treatment effect. It would also make it more difficult to deny the existence of the expected treatment effect even if none is found.

References

1. Fleiss JL: Statistical Methods for Rates and Proportions. New York, John Wiley & Sons, 1973

2. Halpern M, Rosot E, Gurian J, Ederer F: Sample sizes for medical trials with special reference to long-term therapy. J Chron Dis 21, 13-24, 1968

3. First International Symposium on Exercise Testing and Rehabilitation in Cardiology, 1977. Cardiology 62

23
TWO CONSIDERATIONS OF RANDOMIZED CLINICAL TRIALS

Lloyd D. Fisher, Ph.D.

This paper addresses two topics that bear upon the desirability and feasibility of a collaborative clinical trial for the physical conditioning and rehabilitation of myocardial infarction patients. The first topic is the relative benefits of a single site study versus a multiple site (i.e., collaborative) study. Secondly, the analysis problems resulting from nonadherence to a treatment modality (e.g., exercise training) are given. Many important points not considered in this paper may be found elsewhere.[1-3]

Single Versus Multiple Site Studies

The effect on timeliness and numbers of subjects recruited

A study involving multiple sites, when compared to a single site study, has the potential for recruiting more subjects in a fixed time interval or recruiting a fixed number of subjects in a shorter time interval.

Patient recruitment almost always presents severe problems in clinical trials.[4-9] A collaborative study is usually preferable to a single site study that estimates it can barely reach a reasonable number of patients. Peto, et al.[1] point out the many drawbacks of the common study with too few cases.

If a fixed number of subjects are recruited in a shorter time interval, a study will be finished sooner. For many important problems of medical treatment, this is a strong motivation for collaborative research. If the recruitment period is fixed, additional subjects will give added statistical power in detecting treatment differences. Equivalently, if there are more subjects, there are more endpoints (statistical power) in a shorter followup period. However, if it is thought that the response to therapy may vary greatly depending upon the time from treatment, one would still need to follow even a large study for a longer time.

The patient recruitment benefits are lessened by the fact that collaborative clinical trials usually have a longer startup time than a clinical trial carried out at an individual site. This results because it is necessary to recruit the collaborating centers and to standardize the procedures and techniques of the research. Further, some sites may not work as hard at recruiting individuals for the study as they would if the project were under the sole control of the principal investigator at the clinical site. Nevertheless, by having more than one site one may generally recruit a fixed number of subjects faster, or recruit more subjects during a given time period. Experience has shown time and again that it is wise to have an estimate that more subjects can be enrolled than are needed; patient recruitment invariably falls short of even the most pessimistic estimates.

Applicability of the results

One of the difficult problems of science is deciding how broadly inferences may be drawn from a particular study. No matter how well a study is done, it cannot include the population of immediate interest (if for no other reason than that the study was done on last year's patients, while a clinician must treat this year's patients). Depending upon the research, one may have more or less faith in extending the results from one setting to another setting.

In short-term drug studies involving basic physiology, one is more ready to extend findings than in studies involving exercise training. For example, it may be possible to achieve adherence to a training program in suburban or rural areas, but not in urban areas. It may be that adherence is closely associated with socioeconomic variables and/or psychological profiles. In a study involving multiple collaborating sites with varying patient populations, such questions may be investigated if appropriate baseline data are available. It may be that the study method works well in one sociological setting but would not apply in other settings. Even after years of experience, individuals participating in collaborative research are amazed at the amount of variability between clinical sites.

310

Another example: suppose that the particular therapeutic intervention requires great physician skill. One might find in the context of a collaborative study that the method worked well in a few centers but not so well in most other centers. Collaborative research leaves open the possibility of such investigations. Research done at a single institution may have a finding at one extreme, but fail to alert readers to the fact that the center where the study was done is atypical.

Standardization and quality assurance

It is a "truism" to say that one of the weaknesses of collaborative research is the difficulty of developing and maintaining standardized procedures between clinics. Roth and Gordon (1979) contains a series of papers related to standardization and quality assurance.[10-15] Anyone who has been involved in such collaborative research agrees that it is difficult to standardize between clinics. In some ways this represents a strength rather than a weakness of collaborative research. The benefits of such standardization are described below.

During the design phase, it is not unusual for one or more principal investigators to state that a given technique is performed uniformly and reproducibly throughout the country. In many collaborative studies, such statements have been tested empirically and have often proved to be false. For this reason, collaborative studies often go to central evaluation and reading of data, training programs, etc.

Had the principal investigators in a collaborative study been doing their own study, the assumption would be that the given technique was uniform throughout the country. Suppose one or more of the clinics performed their own single site study. Each clinic would proceed in its routine manner. If the results were published, it would appear as though each site were doing the same study. The problem is that clinicians throughout the country read the literature as if the research site performed the "standard" methodology in the same way as it is done at the physician's clinic. Because of lack of detailed knowledge about the methodology, the reading public is led to a false sense of security. A famous physicist once said that we could use π for everything, if we only understood each other. This approach is attempted in the scientific literature. Unfortunately, we do not always know what π stands for.

By contrast, in collaborative studies the collaborators must thrash out numerous details. This usually results in detailed instructions given in manuals of operations. One potential gain from collaborative research is a description of the methodological difficulties with publication of the common methodology. Such gains accrue from collaborative research only if the investigators take the time to communicate with the scientific community.

There is also an educational benefit to the participants in collaborative research. Often this involves formal training about the common methodology. Collaborative research results in additional communication within the scientific community.

There are also drawbacks in collaborative studies. There is a considerable cost both in time and dollars associated with such collaborative endeavors. Mainland[16] suggests that a year for planning and writing a clinical trial protocol, involving at least 100 hours of meetings, is appropriate. The communication and education involved in the collaborative research almost demands that the investigators meet together; this results in expenditures of time and money.

Amount and type of data collected

In collaborative research there is a tendency to collect more data than would be the case in a study at a single site. This results from the many people involved. The investigators have different interests and opinions as to the importance of a given variable. It is easy to negotiate a situation where everybody includes his/her own "favorite" data, not realizing the workload in accruing data. The format of the variables collected may be improved due to examination of the proposed data from a wide variety of views. However, the amount of data may become larger than desirable unless there is clear and powerful direction at appropriate stages of the study design.

Quality of data

The highest quality data result from an excellent study done at a single site. It is not realistic to assume that all published studies result from the highest scientific standards. In collaborative research the average quality of the data tends to be higher. This partially results because there is usually a separate body looking at the data from the individual sites.[14] This monitoring body assesses the timeliness of data submission and the quality of the data. There is external pressure for good performance. Another reason for quality data is that within a collaborative study there is a sharing of knowledge and methodology. This makes available a natural pool of consultants for each site. An

important further reason that collaborative research often results in quality data is that it is often backed
up by considerable funds. This opinion about the quality
of data in collaborative research does not hold if the
individual sites all make the assumption that they are
recording things in the same way. In that case the data
are a hodgepodge of different methodologies and are
probably representative of what appears in the literature, being neither better nor worse than the sites
involved.

Data analysis and publication

In collaborative studies there is a multiple input
during the analysis of study data. This is useful in
detecting weaknesses of analyses. Many of the benefits
of the refereeing system result naturally at an early
stage in collaborative research. However, there is a
danger that the necessity for consensus might downplay
unexpected but strong findings in data.

Collaborative research tends to be slower in analysis
and publication. Several factors contribute to this.
The data will be processed in one place, while the majority of the clinical investigators may be physically
separated. Many of the individuals involved in the data
analysis will not have a sharp awareness of the amount
of work necessary. By being physically separated from
the people doing the analysis there is a possibility
of doing too many analyses or too much manipulation of
the data for little scientific gain. The necessity of
communicating through the mail with drafts of publications adds more time lag. It is easier to spur individuals to immediate action if one may speak to them
face to face.

Expense

Collaborative research is expensive in several ways.
The most obvious expense is money. As discussed above,
the need for standardization and quality assurance results in travel, training sessions for uniformity and
reproducibility of technique, production of manuals of
operations, and visits to the different clinical sites
to observe how they are performing.

A second large expense in collaborative research is
the amount of time spent. Principal investigators travel
to discuss the study and the standardization of the
study. There is additional travel for training in the
techniques used. In order to insure that the collaboration works, there is a large amount of communication both
on paper and by telephone. All of this takes the time
of talented clinical investigators.

313

A further expense of the collaborative research is the emotional effort of many talented people. As participating units in collaborative research are often picked by the peer review system, talented individuals participate in such research. There is considerable ability used not only at the clinical sites, but also at the funding agencies. In some cases one might argue that the talent might have been better used if each individual had done his/her "own thing."

Because of the large expense of money, time, and emotional effort, one should only initiate complex collaborative research when the problem to be studied is very important, or if it is of moderate importance and cannot be solved in any other way.

The Human Factor: Adherence

A clinical trial which involves a large degree of human adherence is difficult to conduct. If one is speaking about exercise training, many of the chapters in this book, including Dr. Shephard's, show that this is a matter of concern in conducting a clinical trial of cardiac rehabilitation. The effect of nonadherence upon the statistical analysis is discussed below. Before proceeding to the specific problems, a few general points about statistical analysis are relevant.

Statistical analysis points

The following two comments are well-known but worth repeating:

- No amount of statistical analysis can compensate for most problems in the scientific design of a study or in the quality of data.

- The scientific results of a study are found with more or less confidence. The amount of confidence one has in a scientific result is on a continuum.

Although in terms of organized knowledge it is useful and, indeed, probably necessary to consider results as proved or disproved, there is a continuum of confidence in any given result. As knowledge advances, results that were "known" to be true have often been shown to be false.

For clinical purposes, results that come from random-ized studies are best.[1,17-21] This because randomized studies have the benefits of assuring that comparable groups are used for the comparison of treatment modalities and of making it possible to quantify the probability that the results occurred because of chance rather than a difference in treatments. These two points hold with very few assumptions.

In an observational data analysis, many assumptions are needed before one can quantify the probability that differences are due to chance. A randomized study makes sure that the treatment groups are comparable on the average, even with regard to important variables that are not recorded or known. Such variables might unconsciously affect assignment to therapy in an observational study. If in an observational data analysis such variables are not recorded, there is no way the analysis can take them into account. For these reasons there is more confidence in the result of a randomized study than in a result that comes from an observational data analysis.

Handling of non-compliance in the analysis of randomized study data

In the primary analysis of any randomized study, individuals should be considered as belonging to the group to which they are randomized.[1,2] If an individual is randomized to an exercise regimen but does not follow through, that individual is still part of the exercise group. If an individual is not randomized to an exercise group but decides to exercise on his or her own, that individual is still in the nonexercise group.

If one needs to separate out those who exercise from those who do not exercise in order to show the findings of the study, then the data analysis results from an observational study and not a randomized study. This point is most important: If the findings of a "randomized study" depend upon the fact that individuals are classified according to whether or not they adhere to their therapy, then the findings result from an observational study and not from a randomized study. This means that the scientific inference is much weaker and should carry less force than had a randomized study turned up the appropriate findings. At this point in time, randomized studies, in some circles, carry a certain mystique and appeal. The author strongly believes in the randomized study for evaluating different treatments. Nevertheless, if there is not enough adherence, the analyses may be observational data analyses, and the strengths of randomized studies would no longer apply.

Some of the potential data analysis problems are illustrated in figure 1. In this hypothetical example, individuals were assigned to exercise and nonexercise groups. Out of those assigned to the exercise group, half complied well but half did not. Of those with good compliance,

suppose that the endpoint rate was only one-half of the
endpoint rate of those with poor compliance. One would

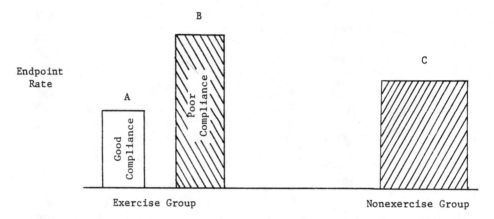

Figure 1. Hypothetical Response of an Exercise Study
with Partial Adherence In the Exercise Group.

think this would indicate a beneficial exercise effect.
Suppose, however, that in the nonexercise group the
rate was precisely that for the combined exercise groups.
If one compared the exercise group to the nonexercise
group, that is, compared A plus B to C, there is no
difference in the endpoint rates. Thus, the data interpretation would be that exercise is not beneficial.

On the other hand, someone may argue that the only
fair comparison group is Group A, who did exercise,
with everyone else who didn't. Thus, one might try to
compare group A, those who actually did exercise, with B
and C. Suppose the result was "statistically significant"
in favor of A, the subset of the exercise group who had
good compliance. Another could counter that the ability
to continue exercising merely split people into high and
low risk subgroups. The argument could go on endlessly.
Some would argue that individuals who drop out or do not
comply with an exercise program do so because prodromal
signs appear, without knowledge being communicated to
those running the study. Further, opponents could argue
that what one really tests in such a trial is the comparison of those who are requested to exercise against those
who are not.[1] There is no overall difference in this
case.

At this point one might then start to analyze the data, looking for the baseline characteristics of the good compliers, as opposed to the poor compliers, and then comparing individuals with the same baseline characteristics in the nonexercise groups. This may or may not be possible depending on the baseline variables collected. The mortality observed could split out in many different patterns. At this point one can see that an observational data analysis is in progress.

From this confusing round of discussion, two principles evolve:

1) The sample size must use realistic dropout rates and assumptions about the effect of that on the endpoint findings.

2) In order to have a strong scientific inference, individuals must be analyzed in the group to which they are randomized, regardless of the subsequent source of therapy. Any other approach reduces the data analysis to that of an observational study rather than a randomized study.

References

1. Peto R, Pike MC, Armitage P, Breslow NE, Cox DR, Howard SV, Mantel N, McPherson K, Peto J, Smith PG: Design and analysis of randomized clinical trials requiring prolonged observation of each patient. I. Introduction and design. Br J Cancer 34:535-612, 1976

2. Peto R, Pike MC, Armitage P, Breslow NE, Cox DR, Howard SV, Mantel N, McPherson K, Peto J, Smith PG: Design and analysis of randomized clinical trials requiring prolonged observation of each patient. II. Analysis and examples. Br J Cancer 35:1-39, 1977

3. Proceedings of the National Conference on Clinical Trials Methodology (Roth H, Gordon RS Jr, eds). Clin Pharmacol Ther 25:no 5, Part 2, 1979

4. Prout T: Patient recruitment: problems and solutions, introduction. Clin Pharmacol Ther 25:679-680, 1979

5. Schoenberger JA: Recruitment in the coronary drug project and the aspirin myocardial infarction study. Clin Pharmacol Ther 25: 681-684, 1979

6. Benedict GW: LRC coronary prevention trial: Baltimore. Clin Pharmacol Ther 25:685-687, 1979

7. Argras WS, Marshall G: Recruitment for the coronary primary prevention trial. Clin Pharmacol Ther 25: 688-690, 1979

8. Croke G: Recruitment for the national cooperative gallstone study. Clin Pharmacol Ther 25:691-694, 1979

9. Prout T: Other examples of recruitment problems and solutions. Clin Pharmacol Ther 25:695-696, 1979

10. Ederer F: Quality assurance of clinical data: introduction. Clin Pharmacol Ther 25:699, 1979

11. Williams OD: A framework for the quality assurance of clinical data. Clin Pharmacol Ther 25:700-702, 1979

12. Kahn HA: Diagnostic standardization. Clin Pharmacol Ther 25: 703-711, 1979

13. Evans JT: Internal monitoring: patient and study management at the clinic. Clin Pharmacol Ther 25:712-716, 1979

14. Mowery RL, Williams OD: Aspects of clinic monitoring in large-scale multiclinic trials. Clin Pharmacol Ther 25:717-719, 1979

15. Ferris FL, Ederer F: External monitoring in multiclinic trials: applications from ophthalmologic studies. Clin Pharmacol Ther 25:720-723, 1979

16. Mainland D: The clinical trial--some difficulties and suggestions. J Chron Dis 11:484-496, 1960

17. Fisher RA: The Design of Experiments, 7th Ed. New York, Hafner Publishing Co, 1971

18. Hill AB: Principles of Medical Statistics, 9th Ed. New York, Oxford University Press, 1971

19. Cox DR: Planning of Experiments. New York, John Wiley, 1958

20. Byar DP, Simon RM, Friedewald WT, Schlesselman JJ, De Mets DL, Ellenberg JH, Gail MH, Ware JH: Randomized clinical trials: perspectives on some recent ideas. New Engl J Med 295:74-80, 1976

21. Chalmers TC, Block JB, Lee S: Controlled studies in clinical cancer research. New Engl J Med 287:75-78, 1972

SUMMARY: PART 6

Michael B. Mock, M.D.

The report of Dr. Charles Francis emphasized the results
of a questionnaire he mailed to 250 physicians in the
greater Hartford, Connecticut area. Although we must
be cautious in any conclusions we draw from a poll with
only a 24 percent response, it does highlight some of the
current physician attitudes of this field. Since the
most commonly reported reason for patient referral for
physical conditioning and rehabilitation was triggered
by the patient's recent myocardial infarction, the potential impact of a large randomized trial in the United
States and Europe on postmyocardial infarction patients
is apparent.

Although 82 percent of Dr. Francis' respondents stated
that they recommend prescribed physical conditioning following a myocardial infarction, it is surprising that the
majority of the same respondents felt that it has no effect on mortality or subsequent cardiac contractility.
Fifty percent of his respondents did feel that the physical rehabilitation program may significantly decrease
morbidity. A rigorously controlled sampling of physicians' attitudes concerning physical conditioning and
rehabilitation would be of value. Recently, Dr. Chalmers
has reported that preconceived attitudes concerning a
therapy may prejudice a physician's interpretation of
the results of a randomized clinical trial. It was encouraging to hear that Drs. Wenger, Hellerstein, and
Blackburn have recently resurveyed approximately 6,000
physicians around the country in terms of their perception of the kinds of needs for rehabilitation of post MI
patients. If their repeat survey has the same 70 percent
reponse reported from their initial survey in 1970, we
will be able to place a considerable amount of confidence

in their interpretation of what has happened to physicians' perception of physical conditioning and cardiac rehabilitaion over the past decade.

Dr. John Naughton, chairman of the steering committee of the National Exercise and Heart Disease Project (NEHDP), reported on the five-center clinical trial sponsored by the Rehabilitation Services Administration. He described the project from its conception in June 1972. The original design called for a definitive clinical trial in which up to 4,300 myocardial infarction patients would be randomized and then followed for up to 7 years. Subsequent funding limitations precluded such an optimal study and mandated a study of lesser scope, which permitted a study of 651 patients between 1973 and 1979.

The protocol for this study called for a low-level physical conditioning program for all referred patients prior to their randomization assignment to either a continued higher level exercise program of physical conditioning or to a control group. The analysis of the results of the initial low-level testing for all referred patients revealed that with their 14 exercise sessions, even though they were of low intensity, were sufficient to produce definite cardiovascular training effects. At the time of randomization, those patients in the exercise training group had a mean aerobic capacity of 7.8 MET's and the control group 8.0 MET's. Eight weeks later the exercise training group subjects showed an increase to 8.6 MET's while the control group remained unchanged. In the ensuing 6 months, the exercise training group experienced only a modest increase in aerobic capacity while the control group showed a decrement. From the 1-year point to the completion of the trial, both groups showed a decreased performance.

Because of the small number recruited into this trial and the problems with compliance and adherence, it is unlikely that this study will provide a definitive answer to the effect of supervised physical conditioning on mortality and morbidity following an acute myocardial infarction. This trial can be considered a valuable feasibility study for this type of trial and has provided some answers on the prognostic value of exercise testing in patients following myocardial infarction.

Dr. Roy Shephard reported on the experience of the Southern Ontario Multicentre Exercise Heart Trial. This group of seven centers studied 750 patients for up to 4 years. Their subjects were randomized either to a high intensity endurance exercise program or to a low intensity homeopathic program of recreational exercise. Their endpoints included reinfarction, death, or defection from the study. Dr. Shephard reported high numbers of dropouts and noncompliers with the exercise program as was reported for the U.S. study. He further reported that despite their recruitment of the stipulated 750 patients, their study will fall far short of the number of specific endpoints (56 valid incidents in the low intensity exercise group and 28 valid incidents in the high intensity exercise group) to reach any statistical significance.

Similar to Dr. Naughton's experience, the Canadian group has produced data on the prognostic value of exercise tests following infarction. Dr. Shephard reported that his study has data that suggest that more than 0.2 mm segmental depression during exercise may increase the chance of a fatal recurrence in patients. He suspected that exercise improved the quality of life of many of the patients enrolled in his study, but admitted that the study has produced no documentation for this belief.

Dr. Veikko Kallio reported on a number of small controlled studies on the cardiac effects of physical exercise from Europe. He reported that, in general, these studies had several problems with adherence to the exercise programs in spite of good protocols and facilities and special arrangements. No conclusive results could be reported from the studies. The major portion of his presentation was a report on the World Health Organization's (WHO) coordinated study. He reported that the WHO Coordinated Study on Rehabilitation and Comprehensive Secondary Prevention in patients after acute myocardial infarction recruited patients between 1973 and 1978. This study was launched to assess the effectiveness of a comprehensive rehabilitation program for reducing recurrent acute myocardial infarction and cardiovascular mortality following an acute myocardial infarction.

In this international effort, major emphasis was given to standardization of evaluation methods and measurements. The major endpoints were death, morbidity (re-infarction, cardiac failure, etc.), and the subsequent number of hospitalizations and the number of days spent in a hospital. Although the study was not planned as an international standardized controlled clinical trial with a common protocol, pooling of some data is possible. The study resulted in 1,630 patients being randomized to an intervention program and 1,488 patients randomized to a control group. In this broad all-inclusive rehabilitation program, the percentages of patients participating in a supervised physical training program at 1, 2, and 3 year followups in the intervention group were 44.8, 37.3, and 30.4 respectively.

In the control groups for the same period, 1.7, 3.4, and 2.1 percent were participating in supervised physical training. In nonsupervised physical training, the percentages for the intervention group were 79.4, 77, and

72.8 and in the control group 61.5, 58.3, and 58.9, respectively. Dr. Kallio pointed out that the high percentage of patients in the control group participating in nonsupervised exercise indicates how popular physical exercise has become in Europe following acute myocardial infarction.

Dr. Kallio reported on the endpoint results of the Finnish portion of this study. They studied 375 consecutive patients from two Finnish cooperating hospitals. Following their discharge from the hospital after a verified myocardial infarction, 188 patients were assigned to the intervention group and 187 to the control group. After 3 years of followup, the total mortality in the intervention group was 20.8 percent, compared to 29.9 percent in the control group. The difference between these two groups is not significant. However, the cumulative coronary mortality in the intervention group was 17.5 percent and sudden death 5.5 percent. The coronary mortality in the control group was 29.4 percent and sudden death 14.4 percent. Thus, there is a significantly smaller number of coronary deaths and sudden deaths in the intervention group compared to the control group. Dr. Kallio concluded that the results of the two Finnish centers suggest that patients with acute myocardial infarction would benefit from an organized comprehensive rehabilitation and intervention program. He could define no single factor responsible for the reduction in coronary mortality and sudden death in the intervention group.

In the discussions of a sample size to show the effect of an exercise program in reducing subsequent mortality following an acute myocardial infarction by at least 33 percent, it was estimated that 3,600 patients would be required. Dr. Shephard stated that this concurred with calculations using the preliminary data from his study indicating a requirement for 4,200 patients.

In the discussion of the ideal endpoints for such a study, Dr. Oberman pointed out that although it is apparent that mortality is the most important endpoint, its use greatly increases the necessary sample size. Dr. Oberman further emphasized the importance of cardiovascular endpoints such as ventricular graphic performance studies determined by echocardiography and angiography, and radionuclide techniques. It was pointed out, however, that although these tests hold great promise, further refinement and evaluation of these as tools to measure the effects of physical conditioning programs on cardiac function remain necessary, particularly for measuring small changes that might result from controlled interventions. It was estimated that the intra- and interobserver variation of the radionuclide techniques

to evaluate ventricular function is in the range of 3 to
5 percent, which is similar to the angiographic techniques. Dr. Oberman emphasized further that the tools
for evaluating the psychosocial effects of exercise also
require refinement.

Dr. Lloyd Fisher reported on the statistical analysis
of collaborative randomized trials. He stated that for
clinical purposes, results that come from randomized
studies are best. This results from the randomization
process assuring that comparable groups are used for the
comparison of the treatment modalities. This makes it
possible to quantify the probability that the results
occurred because of chance rather than a difference in
treatments. He emphasized that the poor compliance with
the exercise protocol for patients randomized to exercise
programs raises a major problem. Both Dr. Fisher and Dr.
Friedewald stated that in the primary analysis of any
randomized study, the subjects should be considered as
belonging to the group to which they are randomized.
Thus, if an individual was randomized to an exercise
regimen but did not follow that program, he still must
be analyzed as part of the exercise group. Likewise, if
an individual is randomized to the control group but
decides to exercise on his or her own, that individual
still must be analyzed as belonging to the non-exercise
group. If, during the final analysis of the data, it is
necessary to separate out those who exercise from those
who do not exercise in order to show significant findings
of the study, then the data analysis results from an observational study and not a randomized study.

Dr. Fisher came to the important conclusion that if
the findings of a randomized study depend on the fact
that individuals are classified according to whether or
not they adhere to their therapy, then the findings of
the study do not carry the scientific inference of a
randomized study. Dr. Fisher concluded by emphasizing
two important points: 1) that an estimated sample size
for a randomized trial must use realistic dropout rates
in assumptions about endpoint findings; and 2) that in
order to have a strong scientific inference, subjects
must be analyzed in the group to which they are randomized, regardless of the subsequent therapy received.
Any other approach reduces the data analysis to an observational study rather than a randomized study.

It was concluded that at the present time a new
collaborative randomized clinical study of the effects
of clinical exercise programs on morbidity and mortality
in patients with cardiovascular disease is not justified.
Experiences of the ongoing randomized trials in the
United States, Canada, and Europe showed high dropout
rates in both groups randomized to the exercise intervention and control groups; furthermore, there was a low

compliance for those continuing with the exercise program.

On the basis of these reports, it was concluded that
a definitive study would require a sample size of 3,000
to 4,000 postmyocardial infarction patients in order to
have adequate statistical power. It was deemed that
this would result in a disproportionate cost and effort
in relation to the type of data that might finally be
realized. This conclusion was based on the experience
reported indicating that conclusions may well be made on
the result of the patient's actual experience rather
than on randomization assignment because of the compliance problems.

Finally, it was felt that the Finnish experience suggests that the more comprehensive investigation employing
a broader risk factor intervention approach including a
program of physical conditioning may ultimately be more
important in evaluating the effect of a cardiac rehabilitation program on mortality and morbidity following an
acute myocardial infarction.

There is a need for continued research effort concen-
trating on small pilot randomized studies of specific
subgroups of cardiovascular patients to further clarify
the value of physical training and other interventions
of multiple risk factors in innovative programs of cardiac
rehabilitation. Potential methods that may yield promising endpoints for these studies include gated blood pool
scans and other radionuclide techniques and also echocardiography. It was emphasized that there were particular
problems with the echo techniques at the present time
since these studies are most useful during rest. It was
also emphasized, however, that the echocardiographic
techniques are attractive in that repeated studies can
be made without radiation hazard, and this technique
permits cycle to cycle change evaluation. Discussions
also emphasized the particular need for developing better
tests of the psychosocial changes that may occur in
cardiovascular patients as the result of rehabilitation
programs.

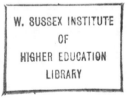